Autoimmune Diet for Beginners

Complete Step-By-Step Guide to Cooking Healthy Dishes and Losing Weight Quickly With the Autoimmune Diet

Alexander Great

described as a work of fiction. Regardless of the nature of this work, the Publisher is exempt from any responsibility of actions taken by the reader in conjunction with this work. The Publisher acknowledges that the reader acts of their own accord and releases the author and Publisher of any responsibility for the observance of tips, advice, counsel, strategies and techniques that may be offered in this volume.

Table of Contents

Chapter 6: Dessert Recipes 152

Conclusion 184

Introduction

Congratulations on purchasing *Autoimmune Diet* for *Beginners*, and thank you for doing so.

The following chapters will discuss the autoimmune diet in greater detail and how it can help you lead a much healthier lifestyle. When people are suffering from autoimmune diseases, the tissues of your body start launching defensive action against your own body, and this causes a lot of damage. But the autoimmune diet or the autoimmune protocol diet, which is also known as the AIP diet, will prevent gut inflammation. The immune system will start to heal slowly, and you will get relief from different autoimmune diseases like rheumatoid arthritis.

It is true that the AIP diet has some similarities with that of the Paleo diet. In this diet, you will be concentrating on eating foods that are rich in important nutrients, and the ultimate goal of the diet is that the autoimmune response from your body's immune system should not be provoked. Once you have successfully started this diet, your gastrointestinal tract will start healing, and the overall inflammation in your body will also be reduced. In short, the diet will mainly be focused on eliminating those foods from your diet that your body is particularly sensitive to.

There are plenty of books on this subject on the
market, thanks again for choosing this one! Every
effort was made to ensure it is full of as much useful
information as possible, please enjoy!

Thanks again for choosing this book, make sure to
leave a short review on Amazon if you enjoy it, i'd
really love to hear your thoughts.

Get the audiobook version of this title
for free with a 30-day Audible trial

Click here if you are from the US:
https://www.audible.com/pd/B08MWSS8CD/?source_code=AUDFPWS0223189MWT-BK-ACX0-221730&ref=acx_bty_BK_ACX0_221730_rh_us

Click here if you are from the UK:
https://www.audible.co.uk/pd/B08MWVLNP1/?source_code=AUKFrDlWS02231890H6-BK-ACX0-221730&ref=acx_bty_BK_ACX0_221730_rh_uk

Click here if you are from the FR:
https://www.audible.fr/pd/B08MWWBXM8/?source_code=FRAORWS022318903B-BK-ACX0-221730&ref=acx_bty_BK_ACX0_221730_rh_fr

Click here if you are from the DE:
https://www.audible.de/pd/B08MWTKN65/?source_code=EKAORWS0223189009-BK-ACX0-221730&ref=acx_bty_BK_ACX0_221730_rh_de

Chapter 1: What Is the Autoimmune Diet?

The autoimmune disease, as stated by many health professionals, is an epidemic. A part of it is thought to be of genetic predisposition, but most of it is because of the eating habits, lifestyle, and the environment. In fact, it is the dietary factors that have been shown to play the most important part in causing autoimmune disease.

What Is the AIP Diet?

This diet is comparatively a newer diet. It consists of a number of food items that are based on the approach of elimination of inflammation from a person's body, which is also the main aim behind this diet. This diet has mainly been created, keeping in mind that the foods will be able to cure the gut. This will ultimately help in reducing the risk of the inflammation that is thought to be created by certain autoimmune conditions.

AIP is the acronym for the autoimmune protocol. This is basically a technique of managing chronic diseases so that the body is provided with the resources of nutrition that is very much required for regulating the immune system, gut health, and healing the tissues while eliminating the stimuli of inflammations from both your lifestyle and diet. This diet gives the body all the nutrients in the exact ratio while eliminating refined and processed foods and those with empty calories. This diet has its own way of encouraging an adequate amount of sleep, managing stress, and other activities that are essential modulators of immunity.

There are basically two ways in which food can be viewed. The first type is the one that enhances good health; for example, the nutrients and the other ones are those that undermine health like those of the inflammatory compounds. The only property that draws a line of distinction between AIP and other dietary measures is that we importantly differentiate between the no foods and the yes foods so that we can fill our pantries with more of the health-promoting compounds and stay away from the detrimental compounds. This is where we choose nutrient-dense foods to say a big no to the compounds that trigger inflammation. This diet is extremely restrictive in nature, eliminating each of those foods that can hold back your health. This diet should not be thought of as a life sentence rather a strategy to know yourself better, to know the ways in which the body will react to a specific food, and at last to know the lifestyle and your surrounding environment.

The Basics of the AIP Diet

- This diet is essentially focused on the elimination of a lot of foods. The goal is to cut the food items or even groups that can trigger inflammation, which can ultimately help in resetting the body's immunity functions. Putting the autoimmune condition into remission and reducing the inflammation in the body will be the idea of this diet that can ultimately be reached by improving eating habits.

- The aim of this diet is to treat a gut that is leaky. This is believed by researchers that those who are suffering from autoimmune diseases mainly have small-sized holes in their intestine. This makes the food get leaked to other parts of the body and triggers the immune system to become reactive. This leaky gut can be healed by eating the foods mentioned in the AIP diet.
- This diet mainly promotes foods that are rich in nutrients and vitamins.

What Are the Benefits of This Diet?

Autoimmune and chronic diseases in our bodies are mainly triggered by the four key areas. Insights that have been drawn on the basis of the information gleaned from twelve hundred studies mainly recommend that this diet and its lifestyle targets that following areas in our body:

- **Gut Health:** Autoimmune diseases are facilitated mainly by a leaky gut or when there is a gut dysbiosis. These two problems have been effectively thought to trigger the development of such diseases. The autoimmune protocol has a list of foods that supports and enhances the growth of various microorganisms that usually grow inside our gut, and they are quite helpful. There are certain foods that cause irritation and, at times, damage the gut lining. These foods are completely struck off from this list mentioned in this protocol. The foods that help the barrier of the gut to improve and restore and also promote the healing of its lining are included in this list. This protocol is also endorsed with the lifestyle factors that are strongly responsible for influencing the health of the gut barrier and also the arrangement of the microbes present in the gut. Gut health is directly linked with the immune function, and if we can restore a healthy gut barrier and the microbiome, then we will necessarily be able to heal them.

- **Immune system regulation:** Regulation of this system is mainly achieved by the restoration of a healthy diversity and by promoting the growth of the healthy microorganisms in the gut. This can also be accomplished by improving the gut barrier function, which can be reached out by providing sufficient quantities of micronutrients that are essential for the normal functioning of the immunity, which in turn will be responsible for controlling the main hormones that keep our immune system in good condition. The foods enlisted in this diet will supply both the opportunity and regulation for the immune regulation. And when the immune regulation gets combined with the process of tissue healing, then this will effectively account for the reduction of the symptoms.

- **Nutrient density:** The various systems in our body, along with the immune system, are mainly run by an array of minerals, essential fatty acids, vitamins, antioxidants, and amino acids. These are essential for the systems to run normally. The key players responsible for the progression of the diseases are the deficiencies in the micronutrient and their imbalances. Consumption of the foods that are dense in the nutrients should be the focus as it enables the cooperative surplus of the micronutrients that are helpful in correcting both imbalances and deficiencies. This, in turn, will be able to support the controlling power of the hormone system, neurotransmitter production, immune system, and the detoxification system. A diet that is filled with nutritious foods is good in providing the body the essential building blocks that are needed to heal the damaged tissues.

- **Hormone regulation:** The types of food that we consume and the time at which we consume them and also the quantity of consumption can affect various hormones that have roles to play in the immune system. Certain dietary factors have been linked to the dysregulation of these hormones that have been found to affect the immune system directly or typically stimulate it. This mainly happens when we consume a lot of sugars or graze on foods instead of eating larger meals with greater time gaps. The diet has been designed in such a way that it promotes the regulation of such hormones, which, in turn, regulates the immune system too. Such hormones are also profoundly impacted by the amount of sleep, or the time we spend outside, the type of activities that we do, and for how long and also by how much we are able to manage our stressful situations.

The most common factor responsible for most of the chronic illnesses is inflammation. This is the only area where changes can be brought by checking up on the foods that we consume. This can make a huge difference in dealing with the problem of inflammation. In certain cases, the immune system can create illness by not able to regulate itself, or in other cases, the inflammation can merely be a component or a contributor to the illness. But inflammation is always considered as the player and the problem. This means reducing the inflammation, and by providing immunity with the resources that it needs, we will be able to deal with the maximum number of chronic diseases. And inflammation can strongly be influenced by the foods we consume and the amount of rest we give to our bodies, how well we can deal with stress, and how much activity we can do. This is why most of us with chronic diseases are able to respond to the diet and lifestyle changes so positively.

Although food cannot be the only cure, still it has certain therapeutic potential for severe illness. Depending on the aggressiveness of the disease, the illness, and how long you have been dealing with it, dietary changes can go a long way in dealing with the problems or may slowly reduce your problems and enhance the quality of living. As we adapt to the foods included in the diet, we become more focused on the consumption of nutrients that support in healing the diseases.

Foods to Include in This Diet

Diet is considered as the core treatment for any kind of disease. It is always given central attention when it comes to treating diseases. Having the proper kinds of food and using this to improve one's health goes hand in hand. Following a diet that is of great use and recommended by professionals and doctors can have immense effects on health, of course, in a good way. This can help the diseases to become non-existent, which, in turn, can ultimately give you a life of unbelievable joy and a tension-free vitality.

Similarly, in this context, we will be focusing on eight such foods that can effectively reduce inflammation and take your tension of dealing with autoimmune diseases away at a go.

Root vegetables

Radishes, carrots, turnips, beetroots, and a lot of other veggies that belong to the family of root vegetables are the staples of this diet. These vegetables can be the best substitute for the grains. The essential nutrients that are found in these vegetables are very crucial in fighting against the diseases that are inflammatory based along with other hazards like heart diseases, diabetes, and cancer. A study that was conducted some time ago in Europe proved that most of the people who included these veggies in their diet were able to solve several problems. They contain healthy carbohydrates, plus they also contain antioxidants and gut-friendly fibers, anti-inflammatory minerals, vitamins, and other nutrients.

Macadamia nuts

These nuts, although they are little-celebrated, and are recessive in the spotlight, still deserve greater attention because of their incredible ways of dealing with detrimental issues. There are free radicals that are neutralized by the antioxidants filled in these nuts, which prevent the damage of cells and other conditions like Alzheimer's disease and diabetes. They boast the greatest levels of flavonoids of all the tree nuts. They help fight against inflammation and to lower bad cholesterol.

They contain both soluble as well as insoluble fibers that can aid digestion and the overall health of the gut. The soluble fibers present in these nuts are capable of acting as prebiotics, which means they can feed the friendly bacteria present in the gut. These bacteria, in turn, produce fatty acids that are short-chained such as propionate, butyrate, and acetate and thus reduces inflammation and protect against diseases like ulcerative colitis, irritable bowel syndrome, and Crohn's disease.

Coconut oil

A lot of skin disorders have a common component, and that is a chronic inflammation, which includes eczema, dermatitis, and psoriasis. And the interesting fact is that coconut oil has certain anti-inflammatory properties that bear with it the power of dealing with these disorders. An experiment was once conducted with rats where coconut oil was applied in their inflamed ears.

Coconut oil was not only able to reduce the inflammation but also relieved them of their pain. They mainly reduced their inflammation by improving the status of the antioxidants and by decreasing oxidative stress. Therefore people with inflammations and autoimmune disease can take a small step for reducing their problems by replacing their cooking oils with coconut oil. It can also add to their taste.

Asparagus

It is a superb source of folate, vitamin C, vitamin B, fiber, and prebiotics. This vegetable is packed with a plethora of nutrients and has its hand, particularly in dealing with the autoimmune diseases because it has a huge quantity of glutathione. This is considered a compound that detoxifies, which breaks down the carcinogens and the free radicals. This, in turn, helps in fighting against inflammation and cancer. Moreover, it also is low in calories, which aid in the loss of weight. It is mainly advised to consume raw as cooking can lead to loss of its nutrients. It is well-balanced with plenty of nutrients, which make it fall in the must-buy list.

Fatty fish

Several oily fishes like mackerel, sardines, and anchovies are a powerhouse for the people suffering from rheumatoid arthritis. In addition to preventing the building up of fat inside the arteries and reducing the blood pressure, consuming these fish can reduce stiffness and joint pains. These fish oils have the properties of anti-inflammation that can treat severe conditions like depression, obesity, heart diseases, and diabetes. Inflammation is a way that is used by our immune system to fight infection and treat several injuries. But chronic inflammation has been connected to these diseases. Consumption of these fish can be a better way of dealing with such disorders.

Avocado

This fruit is the healthiest fruits ever. All thanks to the high content of nutrients in them. They have excellent amounts of antioxidants and monosaturated fats that are healthy. These two factors are equally responsible for dampening the body's inflammatory response. The anti-inflammatory properties of avocados are actually so strong that they can offset unhealthy choices of food. Consuming avocados can lower the triglyceride level of blood, along with a decrease in fat and calories. So when you are consuming this fruit, you are also able to lower your weight as well.

Apple cider vinegar

This vinegar is best known for its anti-inflammatory properties and also has immense health benefits to offer. This vinegar is not only used for cooking but is also connected with various advantages. The properties of reducing inflammation are directly responsible for curing rheumatoid arthritis pain. It has several antioxidants and various other vitamins that aid in making the process go fast. This healthy tonic can aid loss in weight as it can lower the blood sugar level, decrease the level of insulin, reduces the storage of fat, and improves metabolism. It also helps by suppressing the appetite leading to lowered consumption of food.

Olive oil

Diseases of the heart, and other diseases like arthritis, cancer, diabetes are driven by chronic inflammation. Reducing inflammation is the main health benefit of olive oil. Oleic acid that is present in the olive oil mainly acts by reducing the important markers of inflammation. Some of the genes in our bodies are also thought to sometimes drive the inflammation. Olive oil contains such antioxidants that can decrease the numbers of such genes and proteins. It also contains vitamin K and vitamin E in moderate amounts. Thus, it is a package of healthy nutrients that have powerful biological effects.

Chapter 2: Breakfast Recipes

Breakfast Porridge

Total Prep & Cooking Time: Twenty minutes
Yields: One to two servings
Nutrition Facts: Calories: 331 | Carbs: 43.1G | Protein: 7g | Fat: 17.7g | Fiber: 8.7g

Ingredients:

- One cup of squash, chopped and cooked (example: acorn, kabocha or butternut squash)
- Half a cup of coconut milk or water (extra if required)
- One teaspoon of ginger, ground
- Half a teaspoon of cinnamon
- One tablespoon of flaxseed or chia seed (omit for AIP or replace with one tablespoon gelatine powder or collagen)
- Two tablespoons of unsweetened coconut, shredded
- Two to three tablespoons of lightly toasted sunflower seeds (or one tablespoon of tahini) if you can tolerate it. You can use extra two tablespoons of coconut butter (grounded) or coconut flakes as a substitute for seed.
- One pinch each of
- Sea salt
- Turmeric, ground

- Raw honey or maple syrup
- If you're using an Instant pot, you will require additional water and ghee or coconut oil
- Extra toppings: coconut yogurt, coconut cream, pomegranate seeds, cherries, or berries on the top.

Method:

For Stove Top:
1. Mix the dry ingredients (spices, chia seeds, shredded coconut, and sunflower seeds) and grind it in a blender or coffee grinder until you get a flour-like consistency. You can use tahini in place of sunflower seeds if you are short on time and mix them all together.
2. Pour the dry mixture in a small bowl and add the coconut milk or water. Let it absorb and create a gel-like mixture. You can save some of the gel for the topping as well.
3. Add the gel mixture and cooked squash into a blender and blend it until you get a smooth mixture.
4. Cook the porridge on medium heat on a stove-top until it begins to bubble. Stir occasionally.
5. Remove it from the stove-top and pour it into a bowl. Add the dry mixture as a topping.
6. Optional add-in: you can add one teaspoon of ghee if you want. The healthy fats can help absorb the nutrients which improve your digestion and add more nourishment.

7. Add some extra milk, fresh berries as a topping, and serve.

For instant pot,
1. Peel and dice the squash into big pieces. Add one tablespoon of less of coconut oil into the instant pot. Put a pinch of nutmeg and cinnamon and sauté for about five minutes, adding the squash.
2. Pour one-third cup of water into the cooking pot of the Pressure Cooker once the squash is cooked and lock the lid and close the pressure valve.
3. Allow it to cook on Manual High Pressure for about five to six minutes.
4. Give it a ten-minute Natural Pressure Release. If you're short on time, you can also use a quick release. Remove the lid and drain all the water. Then use a hand blender to puree the squash.
5. Combine the remaining ingredients (tahini/sesame mix and the dry mix) and add a splash of milk (non-dairy). Mix everything together. Place the lid back on and let it stay in warm mode until its ready to serve.

Note*: For AIP substitute, you can use seeds if you can tolerate it. You can use coconut flakes or coconut butter combined with some ginger root, grated orange zest, sea salt, and/or cinnamon as a seed substitute in place of tahini or sunflower seeds.*

Turmeric Ginger Lemonade

Total Prep & Cooking Time: Twenty minutes
Yields: Four servings
Nutrition Facts: Calories: 38 | Protein: 0.2G | Carbs: 10.3g | Fat: 0.1G | Fiber: 0.2G

Ingredients:

- Lemon slices
- Juice of one lemon or one-fourth of a cup or more lemon juice
- One to two teaspoons each of
- Ginger or one tablespoon of fresh ginger root
- Turmeric powder
- Two to four tablespoons of raw honey or maple syrup (adjust according to desired sweetness)
- Four to five cups of spring water
- Fresh mint leaves
- Pinch of black pepper to activate the curcumin present in turmeric (optional)
- Stevia for sweetening (optional)
- One teaspoon of lemon powder or lemon extract (optional)

Method:

1. Lightly boil the water on a stove. Add the spices in the water and allow it to boil for another minute. Then reduce the heat and allow it to

simmer for ten minutes. Take it away from the stove and allow it to cool down a little.

2. Pass the liquid through a strainer to eliminate the extra spice powder or ginger root—strain with the help of a cloth or mesh strainer. Pour the remaining liquid into a pitcher and add the sweetener of your choice, lemon juice, and extract. Combine the lemon juice and maple syrup with the turmeric ginger brew properly.

3. Add the fresh mint leaves, extra lemon slices as a garnish, and store it in the fridge. You can add ice if you want, but remember that it will dilute the flavor.

Note*: the beneficial compounds are extracted from the ginger and turmeric by simmering the mixture.*

Bacon and Eggs

Total Prep & Cooking Time: Forty minutes
Yields: Two servings
Nutrition Facts: Calories: 236 | Carbs: 1G | Protein:
19g | Fat: 17G | Fiber: 0g

Ingredients:

- One-eighth teaspoon of ground turmeric
- One tsp of coconut aminos (liquid)
- Two tablespoons of water
- One cauliflower head, diced into four one-inch thick cauliflower 'steaks'
- Six slices of thick-cut bacon (uncured)

Method:

1. Preheat your oven to 400 degrees Fahrenheit.
2. Take a baking sheet and line it with parchment paper.
3. Gently keep the slices of bacon down flat and then place the cauliflower steaks. Make sure that everything is flat on the sheet.
4. Whisk the turmeric, liquid coconut aminos, and water in a small bowl.
5. Gently brush the liquid mixture on top of the cauliflower steaks.
6. Put the baking sheet in the oven and let it bake for twenty minutes.
7. Take it out of the oven, serve, and enjoy!

Matcha Turmeric Latte

Total Prep & Cooking Time: Five minutes
Yields: One serving
Nutrition Facts: Calories: 23.3 | Carbs: 2G | Protein: 0.9g | Fat: 1.3G | Fiber: 0.3g

Ingredients:

- One to two teaspoons of sweetener (honey, maple syrup, coconut sugar)
- One teaspoon of coconut oil
- One and a half cups of milk (non-dairy) (example-almond milk)
- One-fourth of a cup of hot water
- A pinch of black pepper
- One-fourth of a teaspoon of Simply Organic turmeric
- One and a half teaspoons of matcha powder

Method:

1. Take a large mug and add the black pepper, turmeric, and matcha powder into it.
2. Top it with hot water and whisk to combine everything.
3. Heat up the milk so that it begins to froth. Add in the coconut milk and stir it in.
4. Add the milk into the mug and whisk in the sweetener.
5. Drink immediately!

Breakfast Hash

Total Prep & Cooking Time: Twenty-five minutes
Yields: Four servings
Nutrition Facts: Calories: 340 | Carbs: 26g | Protein:
16g | Fat: 17G | Fiber: 4g

Ingredients:

- Eight ounces of spinach
- One and a half teaspoons of extra virgin oil
- Half pound of AIP sausage
- One onion
- Two cloves of garlic
- One large sweet potato
- Coarse sea salt according to taste

Method:

1. Peel the sweet potatoes and chop it into pieces. Remove the sausage from its casing. Peel the onion and chop it. Crush the garlic.
2. Heat a skillet over medium heat. Add the oil and crushed garlic into it and sauté for a minute.
3. Add the diced sweet potato into the skillet and stir.
4. Add in the onion after four to five minutes.
5. Sauté it for about five minutes and stir occasionally.

6. Add in the sausages and break them into pieces
    while stirring it in. Cook it until the sausages
    are no longer pink.
7. Add in the fresh spinach and cook for another
    two to three minutes or until sautéed.
8. Take the skillet away from the heat.
9. Serve hot.

Banana Bread and Carrot Oatmeal

Total Prep & Cooking Time: One hour and ten minutes
Yields: Five to seven servings
Nutrition Facts: Calories: 211.9 | Carbs: 30.1G |
Protein: 4.7g | Fat: 8.6g | Fiber: 2.4g

Ingredients:

- One cup of yellow bananas, mashed (about three medium-sized bananas)
- Thirteen and a half ounces can of coconut milk (full-fat)
- Two ten-ounce bags of shredded coconut
- One-fourth of a cup of coconut flour
- Half a cup of raisins and more for garnishing
- Three-fourth of a cup of unsweetened shredded coconut and more for garnishing
- Two tsp of cinnamon powder
- Two tbsp of liquid honey
- Half a teaspoon of baking soda
- One teaspoon of fine sea salt

Method:

1. Preheat your oven to 350 degrees Fahrenheit.
2. Add all the ingredients in a large mixing bowl and combine them together until all the ingredients are evenly mixed and the shredded coconuts are coated properly.

3. Add the mixture into a nine-inch by thirteen-inch glass casserole dish. Press the mixture down firmly with the help of a spatula. Cover the casserole dish tightly with a foil.
4. Bake it for fifty-five minutes until the oatmeal is still moist, and the carrots are tender.
5. Allow it to cool for five minutes and then serve.
6. You can add some extra coconuts and raisins as a garnish if you want.

Butternut Squash Breakfast Soup

Total Prep & Cooking Time: Thirty minutes
Yields: Two servings
Nutrition Facts: Calories: 220 | Carbs: 34g | Protein:
8.4g | Fat: 7g | Fiber: 7.6g

Ingredients:

- Two medium-sized apples, unpeeled, cored and diced
- One and a half cups of diced butternut squash (frozen)
- Butternut Squash-Apple Blend (about two and a half cups)
- Two tablespoons of plain Greek yogurt (low-fat)
- One tablespoon of pure maple syrup
- One-fourth of a cup of unsweetened plant-based milk or low-fat milk
- A dash each of
- Sea salt
- Ground cinnamon
- One cup of Butternut Squash-Apple Blend
- Filtered water

Method:

1. Add the Butternut Squash-Apple Blend in a large heat-proof bowl. Add water into a medium-sized pot and bring it to a boil. Pour

the hot water over the squash and thaw it. Drain the liquid and then add the squash and apple blend into a high-powered blender. Add about two to three tablespoons of water. Puree it until you get a smooth paste. You can add more water as you feel necessary.

2. You can keep the blend in the refrigerator for three days and in the freezer for up to three months.

3. Heat a pot over low heat. Add the Butternut Squash-Apple Blend along with the other ingredients into the pot until it gets properly warmed and smooth.

Note*: You can sprinkle it with roasted pumpkin seeds or granola if you want.*

Mashed Cauliflower Breakfast Bowl

Total Prep & Cooking Time: Fifteen minutes
Yields: Three servings
Nutrition Facts: Calories: 415 | Carbs: 16.5g | Protein: 21.5G | Fat: 29.2G | Fiber: 4.2G

Ingredients:

- One tablespoon of olive oil
- Two tablespoons of cooking oil (reserve some of the greases for the bacon, you can also use avocado oil, coconut oil, or ghee)
- Three tablespoons of Coconut Aminos (you can also use one and a half tablespoon of balsamic vinegar or three tablespoons of bone broth instead)
- Six to eight slices of bacon
- Four cups of fresh greens
- One and a half cups or one six-ounce package of whole baby Portobello mushrooms
- Half a batch of Ranch Mashed Cauliflower
- Coarse sea salt as a topping
- Sea salt according to taste

Method:

For the mushrooms,
1. Add the cooking oil in a sauté pan and heat it over medium-low heat.

2. Dice the mushrooms in half. Add the diced mushrooms into the pan. Let it slowly cook over low heat so that the flavors fully develop.
3. Pour the Coconut Aminos into the pan when the mushrooms get cooked properly so as to deglaze the pan and add a caramelization on the outer side of the mushrooms.
4. Take the pan away from the heat. While the glaze is still wet, sprinkle some coarse sea salt on top of it.

For the bacon,
1. Preheat your oven to three hundred and seventy-five degrees.
2. Take a rimmed baking sheet and line it with a parchment paper. Lay the slices of bacon on it.
3. Let it bake for twelve to fifteen minutes until it gets crisp.
4. Remove the bacon from the baking sheet and keep it aside on a paper towel to let it cool down a bit. This will help absorb the excess grease. Store the leftover grease present on the baking sheet in an airtight jar in the refrigerator for later use.
5. Roughly chop the bacon once it has cooled down and store it until use.

For assembling,
1. Divide half a batch of the Ranch Mashed Cauliflower and the other ingredients into two

bowls and drizzle a little avocado or olive oil on top of it. Lastly, sprinkle some coarse sea salt on top of it.

2. You can prepare these ingredients a day before and eat it straight out of the fridge or reheat it for a quick breakfast bowl.

**Breakfast Taco Bowls**

Total Prep & Cooking Time: Thirty-five minutes
Yields: Six servings
Nutrition Facts: Calories: 413 | Carbs: 8g | Protein:
22G | Fat: 33g |Fiber: 4g

Ingredients:

For the cauliflower rice,
- One jalapeno pepper, minced
- Twelve ounces of cauliflower rice
- One tablespoon of avocado oil or ghee
- Juice of one lime
- Sea salt and pepper

For the meat,
- One to two tablespoons of broth or water
- One teaspoon of onion powder
- Two teaspoons of taco seasoning (Primal Palate)
- One pound of ground beef
- One tablespoon of avocado oil or ghee
- Sea salt for taste

For the eggs,
- Six large-sized eggs whisked along with two teaspoons of dairy-free milk or water
- One tablespoon of avocado oil or ghee
- Sea salt and pepper according to taste

Additional toppings:
- Minced cilantro for garnishing
- Lime juice
- One avocado, sliced
- Fresh salsa (Pico de Gallo or any other preferred salsa)
- One cup of cherry tomatoes, halved

Method:

For the Cauliflower Rice:
1. Take a large skillet and heat it over medium heat. Once it gets hot, add the avocado oil or ghee. Then add the cauliflower rice and stir to coat it with the oil. Cover the skillet and let it cook for about two to three minutes so that it steams.
2. Remove the cover and stir the rice. Then add the lime juice, salt, pepper, and minced jalapeno pepper to it.
3. Let it cook uncovered for a minute or two, stirring occasionally until you have the desired texture. Then, take the skillet away from the heat.

For the meat:
1. In another skillet or in the same skillet you used to cook the cauliflower rice, add about one tablespoon of avocado oil or ghee and heat it over medium-high heat.

2. Break the beef into pieces and add them to the skillet. Use a spatula or a wooden spoon to break up the lumps.
3. Add the salt and other seasonings into it and cook it. Stir it occasionally and cook until it turns brown. Don't drain the fat.
4. Reduce the heat to medium-low. Then, add the broth or water and combine them together and cook for just enough time so that it gets properly heated. Then, remove it from the heat.

For the eggs:
1. Take a separate skillet and heat it over medium heat.
2. Whisk the eggs properly with the salt, pepper, and milk/water.
3. Add the avocado oil or ghee into the skillet. After the oil gets hot, pour the egg mixture into the skillet and cook over medium heat. Stir to scramble the eggs, and when they are halfway done, reduce the heat to medium-low or low. Scramble the eggs properly over the reduced heat setting until it's cooked to your preference.

Assembling the bowls:
1. Before serving, layer the eggs with the avocados, pico de Gallo, cherry tomatoes, scrambled eggs, and beef.
2. If you're making it ahead of time, you can skip the avocados, salsa, and cherry tomatoes until you're ready to serve.

3. This recipe should make about four to six
    breakfast bowls depending on your appetite.
4. You can add the extra lime juice and cilantro as
    a garnish if you want. Enjoy!

Pumpkin Pie Coconut Parfait

Total Prep & Cooking Time: Four hours and ten minutes
Yields: Four servings
Nutrition Facts: Calories: 271 | Carbs: 12.8g | Protein: 7.8g | Fat: 20.9g | Fiber: 1.8g

Ingredients:

- Half a teaspoon each of
- Mace
- Ground ginger
- One teaspoon each of
- Cinnamon
- Honey or maple syrup
- One tablespoon or one teaspoon of gelatin (it depends on the thickness you want. If you want a Vegan version, use powdered agar instead)
- One cup of pumpkin puree
- One thirteen and a half ounce can of coconut milk (as a coconut-free alternative, you can use two cups of banana milk, tiger nut milk, or homemade coconut milk)

Method:

1. Take a saucepan and add all the above-mentioned ingredients into it. Whisk everything together properly.
2. Heat it until it gets hot to touch.
3. Pour the blend into a glass container.

4. Keep it in the refrigerator for at least four
    hours.

Turkey Apple Breakfast Hash

Total Prep & Cooking Time: Thirty minutes
Yields: Five servings
Nutrition Facts: Calories: 297 | Carbs: 24.1G | Protein: 24.6g | Fat: 12.5G | Fiber: 4.7g

Ingredients:

For the meat,
- Half a teaspoon each of
- Dried thyme
- Cinnamon

- One tablespoon of coconut oil
- Sea salt to taste
- One pound of turkey, ground

For the hash,
- Half a teaspoon each of
- Turmeric
- Dried thyme
- Garlic powder
- Three-fourth of a teaspoon of ginger powder
- One teaspoon of cinnamon
- Two cups of spinach or other greens of your choice
- One large-sized apple, peeled, cored, and diced

- Two cups of frozen butternut squash or sweet potato, diced into cubes
- Half a cup of carrots, shredded
- Two small or one large zucchini
- One onion
- One tablespoon of coconut oil
- Sea salt according to taste

Method:

1. Take a skillet and heat it over medium or high heat. Add one tablespoon of coconut oil into it. When it gets hot, add in the ground turkey and cook it until it turns brown. Add a pinch of sea salt, dried thyme, and cinnamon as the seasoning. Stir everything and then transfer it on to a plate.
2. In the same skillet, add the remaining coconut oil. Add the onions into it and sauté for two to three minutes so that they get softened.
3. Add the frozen squash, apples, carrots, and zucchini. Cook it for about four to five minutes until the vegetables turn soft.
4. Add in the spinach and stir until they get wilted.
5. Add in the cooked turkey, salt, and the other seasonings and stir them together and then turn off the heat.
6. You can keep this hash in the refrigerator and eat it throughout the week or enjoy it fresh from the skillet.

7. The hash can be kept in a sealed container in the refrigerator for about five to six days.

__Note__: You can use fresh quash if you don't have frozen squash. However, it might take longer to cook. You can use your favorite veggies or ground meat. Just remember that the cooking time will need to be adjusted. You can adjust the seasonings as you see fit to your taste.

Sausage Chicken Poppers

Total Prep & Cooking Time: 40 minutes
Yields: Two to four servings
Nutrition Facts: Calories: 107 | Carbs: 1G | Protein: 7g
| Fat: 8g | Fiber: 0g

Ingredients:

- Two to three slices of bacon, finely chopped
- Half a cup each of
- Apple, finely diced
- Spinach, finely chopped
- One cup of sweet potato, shredded
- One pound of chicken or turkey, ground
- One teaspoon each of
- Rosemary
- Ground sage
- Two tablespoons each of
- Coconut oil
- Coconut flour
- Half a teaspoon of sea salt

Method:

1. Preheat your oven to 400 degrees Fahrenheit.
2. Take a baking sheet and line it with parchment paper.
3. Take the shredded raw potato and remove the excess water from it by squeezing it with the help of a cheesecloth or paper towel.

4. Add the bacon slices, apple, spinach, sweet potato, and chicken in a large mixing bowl and mix them properly to combine everything together. The shredded sweet potatoes are the primary base of the poppers. You can skip the bacon if you want, but it increases the flavor and gives more of a breakfast feel to these sausage poppers. The texture and flavor of the spinach are not overpowering and harsh, so it helps add some nutrients to the poppers and works best in this recipe. The apple in the sausages adds an awesome flavor to it. Among apples, pink lady and granny smith variety work best, but you can also use other varieties.

5. Then, add the seasonings, salt, coconut oil, and coconut flour into the mixing bowl and combine everything together. The coconut oil and coconut flour will help bind all the ingredients together and make them crispier. Although coconut flour produces the best flavor, you can substitute them with other flours like almond or cassava flour if you want.

6. Start rolling the mixture into tiny portions about an inch in diameter and slightly flatten each portion with the palm of your hand. You will get around twenty to twenty-five poppers. Transfer them onto the baking sheet.

7. Let it bake it in the oven for approximately twenty-five to twenty-eight minutes. Flip them halfway through.

8. If you want you can make the poppers even crispier, you can cook them under the broiler or in a pan for one to two minutes.
9. When they are cooked thoroughly, remove them from the oven.
10. Let the poopers cool down and serve immediately. You can also make them ahead of time and store them in the freezer or refrigerator as a make-ahead breakfast.

Note: *All the ingredients that are mentioned are raw.*

Butternut Breakfast Bites

Total Prep & Cooking Time: Three hours
Yields: Four to five servings
Nutrition Facts: Calories: 105 | Carbs: 7g | Protein: 5g
| Fat: 6g | Fiber: 1G

Ingredients:

- One cup of cooked butternut, mashed
- One pound of lamb (or beef or pork), ground
- Three tablespoons of freshly chopped parsley
- Ten mint leaves (if you are using lamb) or cilantro or coriander (if you're using pork or beef), finely chopped
- One teaspoon each of
- Garlic powder
- Sea salt
- Half a teaspoon of cinnamon powder

Method:

1. Preheat your oven to 200 degrees Celsius or 400 degrees Fahrenheit.
2. Take a large mixing bowl and add the mashed butternut, ground lamb, finely chopped mint leaves, cinnamon, garlic powder, and sea salt and mix everything together with the help of your hands so that the butternut and the spices are properly combined with the meat.

3. Roll this mixture into one and a half-inch balls with the help of your hands or a small cookie scoop and keep these balls in mini muffin tins.
4. Keep the muffin tins in the oven and let it bake for twenty minutes until the meat is no longer pink and the edges have turned golden brown.
5. Remove the balls from the muffin tins and serve hot.

Tapioca Porridge

Total Prep & Cooking Time: Forty-five minutes
Yields: Three servings
Nutrition facts: Calories: 352 | Carbs: 58.1G | Protein: 3.8g | Fat: 12.8g | Fiber: 7.3g

Ingredients:

- For the raspberry-rhubarb sauce,
- One packet of Stevia powder (or according to your preference)
- One cup of raspberries
- One tablespoon of water (or as required)
- Two cups of frozen rhubarb (chopped)
- One teaspoon of coconut oil
- For the porridge,
- One tablespoon each of
- Vanilla extract
- Maca powder (for example, Organic Burst)
- Two dates, pitted and chopped
- Two-third of a cup of coconut milk
- Three-fourth of a cup of small tapioca pearls
- Two cups of water (or as required)
- One packet of Stevia powder (or as required)

Method:

1. Take a saucepan and grease it with coconut oil. Keep the pan over medium heat and add the

rhubarb. Cook the rhubarb for about ten minutes until it gets soft. Add water if required.

2. Add the packet of stevia powder and raspberries and stir it into the rhubarb. Cook for five to ten minutes until the sauce gets smooth.
3. Take a pot and fill it halfway with water. Bring it to a boil and then add the tapioca. Let it simmer over medium heat for about a minute, stirring occasionally. Decrease the heat to low and keep stirring for five to eight minutes until the tapioca turns completely translucent.
4. Take a blender and add the vanilla extract, maca powder, dates, and coconut milk into it. Blend until you get a smooth paste.
5. Use a fine-mesh strainer to strain the tapioca porridge. Keep the pot over low heat and transfer the strained tapioca back into it. Add in the packet of stevia powder and coconut mixture into the porridge and stir it in.
6. Let it simmer for five more minutes until all the liquid is absorbed.
7. Transfer the porridge into three wine glasses and add the raspberry-rhubarb sauce as a topping.

Carrot Cake Breakfast Cereal

Total Prep & Cooking Time: Fifteen minutes
Yields: Two servings
Nutrition Facts: Calories: 383 | Carbs: 45g | Protein: 11G | Fat: 14g | Fiber: 10g

Ingredients:

- Half a cup each of
- Apple cider (or, unfiltered apple juice)
- Finely grated carrots (one medium-sized carrot)
- Two cups of spaghetti squash, cooked
- One-fourth of a cup of coconut milk (full-fat)
- Two tablespoons of raisins
- One-fourth of a teaspoon of ground ginger
- Half a teaspoon of cinnamon
- One teaspoon of vanilla
- Toppings (optional):
- Chopped nuts (skip if you're following elimination-stage AIP)
- Shredded carrot

Method:

1. Take a saucepan and add all the ingredients (except the nuts and raisins) and mix them together and bring to a gentle simmer. Let it simmer for five to seven minutes until the mixture gets thick.

2. Process a couple of times with the help of a hand-held blender to achieve a porridge- or oatmeal-like consistency.
3. Add in the raisins and let it simmer for about a minute or two.
4. Remove from the heat and serve. Add the toppings and an extra drizzle of coconut milk as a garnish if you want.

Chapter 3: Lunch Recipes

Sardines and Baked Sweet Potatoes

Total Prep & Cooking Time: 1 hour 10 minutes
Yields: Four servings
Nutrition Facts: Calories: 220 | Carb: 29.1G | Protein: 13.6G | Fat: 5.5g | Fiber: 4.1G

Ingredients:

- Four medium-sized sweet potatoes
- One medium, thinly sliced, red onion
- Two cloves of garlic, plump (minced)
- One tablespoon each of
- Oregano (chopped finely)
- Lard (solid fat), you may include some extra for adding in the potatoes
- Half a bunch of green kale, chopped roughly
- A handful of small parsley, flat (chopped)
- Five ounces of chopped brown mushrooms
- Six anchovy fillets (rinsed properly, from the can)
- Half a cup of pitted olives, green and chopped
- Two cans of sardines (packed in olive oil or spring water and drained

Method:

1. Set the oven at a temperature of 400 degrees F. Pierce the sweet potatoes for a number of times. Take a baking sheet (possibly a large one) and then lay the pierced potatoes on the sheet. Bake the potatoes for one hour. You may even need to bake it more or less depending on the potatoes' size.
2. While the potatoes are getting baked, utilize the time by placing a sauté pan (large-sized) on another oven to heat it. Add the fat (lard) in the pan. Sprinkle the chopped onion pieces in the pan and then make the whole thing warm by allowing it to cook for about six to eight minutes. By this time, the fat must get translucent and become soft.
3. Increase the flame to medium and then in the pan, place the chopped mushrooms, stir them properly for about three to four minutes so that they get coated with the fat, and their edges become brownish.
4. Add the oregano, anchovies, and minced garlic one by one into the pan and give another two minutes to get them cooked.
5. Now you may add the kale and olives to sauté pan and then cook for about four minutes until you notice the kale to form wilts and add sardines to it after that. Warm through the entire thing. Use a wooden spoon to break them into large mouthful pieces.
6. Finally, throw the parsley in the pan and mix everything to incorporate.

7. Make splits in the potatoes up to its middle (lengthwise). In the groove, place a lump of solid fat. Do this for all the potatoes and top each of them with the prepared sardine mixture.
8. Serve this hot and spicy dish immediately.

Note: You must be aware of the source of the olives. Some of them are stuffed into brines that contain citric acid and lactose that are not at all AIP-friendly.

Creamy Cauliflower Noodles

Total Prep & Cooking Time: 50 minutes
Yields: Eight plates of noodles
Nutrition Facts: Calories: 344 | Carbs: 7g | Protein: 4g
| Fat: 35g | Fiber: 1G

Ingredients:

The cauliflower,
- One large-sized cauliflower head (the head should be sliced into small florets)
- One tsp. each of
- Garlic (granulated)
- Sea salt
- Two tbsp. of avocado oil
- *For the noodles,*
- Veggie noodles of your choice

For preparing the sauce,
- Three cups of fresh basil (Thai, regular or purple)
- A cup each of
- Avocado oil
- Cashews water-soaked and then drained
- Half a tsp. of fine salt
- Three garlic cloves
- Two tsp. of fish sauce
- One tbsp. of lemon zest

Method:

1. Keep the oven preheated to a temperature of 400 degrees Fahrenheit.
2. In a small-sized bowl for mixing, add florets of cauliflower and along with it some drops of oil, the minced garlic, and sprinkle some salt. Toss them very well to coat properly and then lay them out evenly on a casserole dish. Roast the florets for about thirty-five minutes and notice their color to become a bit brownish.
3. Meanwhile, use all the ingredients for the sauce to prepare it. Place the ingredients in the blender, then process. Blend them until they become smooth. Transfer to a blow and set it aside, covered.
4. Cut the packets containing the noodles, and place them in a bowl after draining them properly. Keep the noodles immersed in a bowl full of water and allow it to soak for about five minutes. After that, you may strain the excess water and keep it aside.
5. Keep checking the florets as well. Once you find they have become golden, take them off the oven and then add them to the noodles. With the help of a tong mix everything properly and then again spread them evenly on the casserole dish.
6. Now place the dish in the oven to bake for another fifteen minutes. Transfer to a serving plate and enjoy.

Note: *Cauliflower is known to contain the fibers that are important to feed the good bacteria that are present in the gut, which, in turn, is responsible for reducing inflammation and promote a healthy digestive system functioning properly. When consumed in adequate quantities, these fibers can also aid in improving the digestive conditions like diverticulitis, inflammatory bowel disease, and even constipation. Consumption of these fibers in adequate amounts has been connected to decreased hazards of illnesses, cancer, diabetes, and heart diseases.*

Teriyaki Turkey Meatballs

Total Prep & Cooking Time: 28 minutes
Yields: Six meatballs
Nutrition Facts: Calories: 237 | Carbs: 6g | Protein:
30g | Fat: 11G | Fiber: 1G

Ingredients:

- One tablespoon each of
- Coconut aminos
- Powder of mushroom (optional)
- One teaspoon each of
- Salt
- Onion powder
- Garlic powder
- Half a tablespoon each of
- Apple sauce
- Coconut flour
- Half a teaspoon each of
- Ginger powder
- Fish sauce
- One pound of turkey (ground, dark meat)

Method:

1. Set the oven at a temperature of 350 degrees
    Fahrenheit. While the oven is still on, add the
    apple sauce, garlic powder, fish sauce, coconut
    aminos, onion powder, ginger powder,
    mushroom powder, and salt one after the other

in a large-sized mixing bowl. Mix them well so that they become incorporated properly.

2. Now add the remaining two ingredients-coconut flour and the turkey. Add a pinch of salt again and combine it.
3. Now take some amount mixture in your hand and drift them in the shape of balls of size two inches. Do the same for the total quantity of mixture. This will form around six to seven balls.
4. Take a sheet pan and grease it properly. Lay down the balls on it.
5. Bake the meatballs in the oven that has been preheated, for about twenty minutes.
6. Serve the meatballs with as much mint or cilantro as you want, along with some avocados. Enjoy!

Note:

- ***Ginger*** *- This vegetable has immense health benefits. Mixing ginger along with tea can help to fight against cold. They help with abdominal issues, vomiting, and nausea. It also helps to prevent certain dangerous disorders like those of tumors, migraines, cancer, diabetes, and ulcers. This can also be utilized in various ways to treat inflammations. They can either be utilized as capsules or as a tincture.*
- ***Garlic*** *- This vegetable is filled with various therapeutic and prophylactic agents. These cloves have the potential of preventing cancer.*

They are also known to increase the strength of the immunity, which is brought by their property that they can reduce inflammation. They have compounds rich in sulfur, which increases the biological activities of this vegetable. This is the main reason why they are used in the treatment of cancer.

Roasted Chicken Thighs

Total Prep & Cooking Time: 1 hour 10 minutes
Yields: Two plates
Nutrition Facts: Calories: 336 | Carbs: 2G | Protein:
31G | Fat: 21G | Fiber: 0g

Ingredients:

- One teaspoon each of
- Avocado Oil
- Gyro seasoning (primal)
- Twelve garlic cloves (unpeeled and one full fist)
- Pinch of pink salt (Himalayan)
- Four chicken thighs (skinned)

Method:

1. Set your oven at a temperature of 350 degrees F.
2. Turn the flame of the oven to medium heat and then place a medium-sized pot in it. Pour the avocado oil and the cloves of garlic inside the pot and sauté the whole thing for two to three minutes. This must bring garlic skins to a brownish tinge.
3. Use another oven to place a large-sized skillet and turn the flame to moderate to strong heat. Sear the thighs of the chicken on both sides. The side that has the skin must be done first to prevent the pieces from getting stuck in the

skillet. This can be done for three minutes for each side.

4. Now you may add chicken thighs to the pot where the garlic was kept sautéed and sprinkle with gyro seasoning and add a pinch of the pink salt. Blend them well to form a well-coated mixture of all the ingredients. The mixture, after getting incorporated, must be baked for about an hour after covering up the whole thing.

5. Transfer to the serving plate and fill the faces of the plate with the vegetables of your choice.

***Note:** Chicken is usually considered as a healthy yet lean protein, which has some amount of good fat that makes it to have the overall nutrition. Therefore it is important to use skinned chicken, plus it also makes it yummy. The main factor that makes its sure-shot inclusion in this recipe is that it is an anti-inflammatory food. Which means it can reduce the inflammation that is believed to be the core cause of autoimmune diseases. Including chicken in the diet can actually aid you in managing your disease well. This is a food that is considered to be very important and always preferred by health professionals as well.*

Feel Good Soup

Total Prep & Cooking Time: 30 minutes
Yields: Two bowls
Nutrition Facts: Calories: 294 | Carbs: 5g | Protein:
23G | Fat: 16g | Fiber: 1G

Ingredients:

- One tablespoon of coconut oil
- Six cloves of garlic (minced)
- One teaspoon of Pink salt (Himalayan)
- Two tablespoons each of
- Coconut vinegar
- Nutritional yeast (optional)
- A quarter cup of coconut cream
- Three fists full of baby spinach
- Two to four collagen peptides (optional)
- Two cups of sliced mushrooms (cremini)
- Three springs of thyme
- One cup each of
- Bone broth
- Riced cauliflower

Method:

1. Place a pot of medium size over moderate
   flame and pour the coconut oil. Bring it to a
   boil, and then you may add the seasonings,
   thyme, mushroom, and the garlic.

2. Occasionally stir the mixture in the pot, unless you are able to smell the aroma, and everything gets wilted, stirring them for eight minutes or so.
3. Deiced the pot by adding the coconut vinegar. Scrap up anything that you will find stuck at the sides of the pot.
4. And now you may add the cream of coconut and the bone broth. Put the oven to simmer and let it cook.
5. Now you will stir in the spinach and cauliflower rice. Allow these two to become tender for five minutes in the pot. Then add the peptides and, finally, the yeast. Cook until they get dissolved. Serve in a bowl and enjoy.

Note: *Coconut oil is essentially considered as the best anti-inflammatory food as it tops the list and also because it has been proved. It is packed with vitamins and minerals, and it has the goodness of fiber and some of the important antioxidants. It is mainly used as a substitute for canola oil and corn oil as these oils can destroy the cells, specifically in those who are suffering from autoimmune disease.*

Chicken Shawarma Salad

Total Prep & Cooking Time: 30 minutes
Yields: Two bowls of salad
Nutrition Facts: Calories: 716 | Carbs: 18g | Protein: 51G | Fat: 49g | Fiber: 4g

Ingredients:

For the chicken pieces,
- Two breasts of chicken, sliced into small cubes
- One tbsp. each of
- Garlic powder (approximately ten grams)
- Onion powder (approximately seven grams)

To taste: Salt
- One tsp. of turmeric (approximately two grams)
- Half a tsp. of oregano, dried (approximately one gram)
- Four tbsp. of avocado oil (approximately sixty milliliters)

For the salad dressing,
- Two tbsp. of olive oil (approximately thirty milliliters)
- Salt
- One tbsp. of lemon juice (approximately fifteen milliliters)

For the salad,

- Two cups of washed salad leaves
- One sliced beetroot, pickled
- Parsley for the purpose of garnishing
- One sliced cucumber
- Half an onion sliced

Method:

1. Prepare the dressing for this recipe by combining the lemon juice and the olive oil (as per the quantities mentioned in the ingredients section). Mix them in a small-sized bowl and season them with salt. Mix them properly with a spoon, and then keep it aside.
2. In another bowl, mix the garlic powder, turmeric powder, oregano, and the onion powder. Sprinkle some amount of salt and mix them. Then drop the pieces into the mixture and coat them.
3. Put the frying pan on the oven on moderate heat and pour a few drops of the avocado oil. Drop the coated chicken pieces in the pan. Cook them carefully, turning the sides to cook evenly. Remove the pieces from the oven and then place them on a plate.
4. Alternatively, the spiced chicken pieces may also be skewed onto a kebab stick and then grill. Gently remove the pieces from the sticks.
5. Now it is time to prepare the salad. You will require a bowl to prepare it. You can do that by simply tossing the cucumber and the salad

greens in the prepared salad dressing and placing them inside the bowl. Top this combo with the chicken pieces. Add the beetroot and the onion pieces on top. Crown with parsley leaves to garnish.

Chipotle Chicken Lettuce Wraps

Total Prep & Cooking Time: 40 minutes
Yields: Eight wraps
Nutrition Facts: Calories: 177.2 | Carbs: 4.5g | Protein: 12.7G | Fat: 12.4g | Fiber: 2.4g

Ingredients:

- Two tbsp. of olive oil (divided and extra virgin)
- Two or three chipotle peppers, depending on your love for spicy
- Half a cup of cilantro (freshly chopped)
- One red or yellow or orange bell pepper (sliced)
- One diced avocado
- Salt to taste
- One pound of chicken breast (skinless and boneless)
- Three tbsp. of adobo sauce
- One lime
- Three thinly sliced scallions
- One head iceberg lettuce (washed and the leaves separated)

Method:

1. Turn the oven to moderate heat and place a large-sized saute pan. Pour the olive oil in the pan and boil. Now you may add the pieces of chicken to the pan. Season the pieces with salt and then for about six minutes sear them until

you notice they are cooked thoroughly, and the chicken becomes brownish from all the sides.

2. Then you may transfer the chicken to a board basically used for cutting and then allow it to sit for five minutes. Then cut the pieces into small pieces.
3. Now put the sliced bell peppers to a saute pan and cook for three minutes so that they become soft and then remove them from the pan.
4. Now you will require a food processor to process some of the ingredients. Inside the bowl of the processor, add adobo sauce, lime juice, chipotle pepper, and cilantro. Process them to form a smooth paste.
5. Pour the chipotle sauce you have just prepared into the pan and add the fried and seared chicken into the pan again. Toss them well to coat with the sauce by stirring them properly.
6. Fill the cups of the lettuce with two tbsp. of the mixture of chicken and then garnish with avocados and scallions.
7. Serve and enjoy.

__Note__: Lettuce leaves are packed with effective nutrients that are of great use to the human body. They have properties that help to reduce inflammation and specifically have proteins like carrageenan and lipoxygenase that helps in the reduction of the inflammation. Therefore, lettuce is usually selected by health professionals for those suffering from autoimmune disorders. They are filed with antimicrobial properties, which can help in *controlling the anxiety as they have sedative effects, and because of this property, it can induce sleep. In addition to these properties, these leaves can also make your skin look beautiful because of the presence of a great number of antioxidants in them.*

Stuffed Chicken Breast

Total Prep & Cooking Time: 40 minutes
Yields: Two servings
Nutrition Facts: Calories: 661 | Carbs: 8g | Protein: 50g | Fat: 48g | Fiber: 4g

Ingredients:

- For preparing stuffed chicken breast,
- Half the head of cauliflower, broken into small florets (approximately 300 grams)
- Two chicken breasts (each breast approximately of 200 grams)
- Two tbsp. each of
- Avocado oil (approximately 30 milliliters)
- AIP pesto
- Pinch of salt to taste
- For preparing the AIP pesto,
- One-third cup of olive oil (approximately 80 milliliters)
- Two cloves of roughly chopped garlic
- Salt
- One and a half cups of basil leaves (approximately 50 grams)
- Half a lemon zested and juiced

Method:

1. Add the basil leaves, olive oil, garlic, and the lemon (half of it) zest and juice in a processor to prepare the pesto. Add some more olive oil into the processor if required. Season the entire thing with salt. Two tablespoons of this recipe will only be required, and rest can be easily kept in the refrigerator for up to three days.
2. Set your oven at a temperature of 350 degrees F and keep it preheated.
3. Using the microwave or steamer, cook the florets of cauliflower until they become tender. After they are done, remove and mash the well so that they become smooth. Add two tbsp. of the pesto that you have prepared and stir it well to coat them properly with the paste. Store the pesto coated florets aside.
4. Marinade the chicken breasts using salt. Make incisions on only a particular side of each of the chicken breasts. The cuts must be deep.
5. Turn the oven on and on moderate heat fry the chicken breasts in two tbsp. of the olive oil. Turn the breasts and cook each side properly until they become golden. After they are cooked, transfer them to a work surface. You are required to be careful about the place where you will be keeping the chicken breasts and about the utensils you will be using as the breasts will be fairly raw in the side.
6. After allowing the chicken breasts to become cool, fill the pockets of each of the chicken breasts with the cauliflower-pesto mixture. Place the entire preparation on a roasting tray

and then bake it for another twenty minutes so that the chicken gets sufficiently cooked through.

7. You may serve it with sweet potatoes or your choice of salad.

**Salmon Salad Bowls**

Total Prep & Cooking Time: 30 minutes
Yields: Four bowls of salad
Nutrition Facts: Calories: 470 | Crabs: 10g | Protein: 36g | Fat: 32G | Fiber: 5g

Ingredients:

- Eight cups of romaine lettuce (finely chopped)
- One teaspoon each of
- Paprika (smoked)
- Garlic powder
- Salt
- Four fillets of salmon (the fillets must be of the same size)
- Vegetables as per your choice- cucumber, tomatoes, kraut, carrots
- Black pepper

For the dressing,
- One avocado (remove the peel and get pitted)
- One lemon juiced
- One teaspoon each of
- Apple cider vinegar
- Black pepper (ground)
- One tablespoon of Dijon mustard
- A quarter cup of olive oil
- Half a teaspoon of sea salt
- Three peeled garlic cloves

Method:

1. Set the oven to a temperature of 400 degrees F and keep it preheated, meanwhile, with the help of a parchment paper line the baking sheet.
2. Place the even fillets of salmon over the baking sheet. Season the fillets with garlic powder, salt, pepper, and smoked paprika. Now place the baking sheet in the preheated oven and allow the filets to bake for about fifteen to twenty minutes until you notice that the fillets have become brownish. You should be able to feel the fillets a bit flaky when touched with a fork.
3. The size of the fillets will be determining the cooking time. It may increase or decrease.
4. Chop the romaine lettuce and keep them aside.
5. Preparing the dressing: you will require a food processor to prepare the dressing. Inside the bowl of a processor, add all the ingredients that have been listed in the ingredients section (for dressing) except the olive oil and salt. Start to blend so that everything gets well combined. Now you may add olive oil to the processor slowly while it is still processing to make the paste even more creamy and smooth. Once the paste tastes creamy, you may add the salt as per your taste.
6. Divide the dressing into half and pour one half to the romaine. Toss the leaves well to coat with the dressing properly. Set it aside.

7. You will use the second half of the salad dressing to coat the veggies. This will prepare a great snack. Or you may add them on top of the salad bowls.

8. Remove the salmon fillets from the oven as it should have got cooked by now. Make the salmon fillets into round bowls and fill each of them with romaine. Serve with the coated veggies with an extra spoon of the dressing. Enjoy!

Broiled Salmon

Total Prep & Cooking Time: 28 minutes
Yields: Six plates
Nutrition Facts: Calories: 260 | Carbs: 3g | Protein: 20g | Fat: 18g | Fiber: 0g

Ingredients:

- One and a half pounds of salmon (wild-caught)
- Two tbsp. of olive oil
- Chives for the purpose of garnishing
- One tsp. of salt (fine)
- A quarter cup each of
- Coconut aminos
- Orange juice (freshly squeezed)

Method:

1. If by no means you like to scrub your pan forever, then essentially use a parchment paper to line the sheet pan. Set the pan to some other place.
2. Sprinkle a pinch or two of salt all over the salmon.
3. In a small-sized bowl, add olive oil, coconut aminos, and orange juice and whip them properly to mix well.
4. The prepared marinade will now be used to coat the salmon pieces. For that, you will be required to start by putting down the meat side of the salmon into the marinade.

5. Set the oven to a temperature of 550 degrees F. now use a parchment paper to let the skin side of the salmon to sit on it. And pour the marinade that you have prepared (from orange juice, aminos, and the olive oil.) on the salmon.

6. Place the parchment paper containing the salmon mixture under the broiler. Allow it to cook thoroughly. This will take about eight minutes. It might take some more time. Just notice that the salmon flakes when you insert a fork into it. Once the eight minutes mark is crossed, keep checking the salmon to prevent it from getting overcooked.

7. The chives will now be used to garnish this dish. After you are satisfied with your flaked salmon, transfer it to the serving plate. Place the chives on top of the salmon. Serve it hot to enjoy the best of it.

Note: The immune system of our body uses the response of inflammation as an important part. But excessive inflammation can actually lead to some adverse effects in our system. Salmon fish, as discovered by researchers, contains fatty acids that have been found in suppressing the inflammatory response of our body in a number of ways. Certain chemicals are present in our body that are thought to be pro-inflammatory is mainly responsible for triggering inflammation response. Salmon oil can help reduce such chemicals. Reduction in inflammation can reduce other conditions like heart disease and arthritis and manage the immunity as well.

Lemon Tuna Salad

Total Prep Time: 10 minutes
Yields: One bowl of salad
Nutrition Facts: Calories: 480 | Carbs: 11G | Protein: 45g | Fat: 40g | Fiber: 8g

Ingredients:

- One-third of a cucumber, dice it into medium-sized pieces
- One tsp. of lemon juice
- One tbsp. of olive oil
- Half a small-sized avocado (finely diced)
- One can of tuna (one fifty grams)
- Salad greens (optional)
- Salt

Method:

1. In a bowl, mix the avocado and the cucumber that has been diced along with the olive oil (as per the measurement given in the ingredients section).
2. In the frying pan, put the tuna fish and cook so that it becomes flaky. Then you will have to mix the mustard and the mayo into the flaked tuna.
3. Now it is the time to put the tuna mixed with mustard and mayo into the bowl that had the cucumber and avocado. Add some salt to this bowl over this mixture, and then toss them well.

4. Prepare the salad greens for the purpose of garnishing. In order to do it, mix the greens with oil and the juice from lemon to make it taste better.
5. After the salad greens are prepared, put the tuna salad on top of it.
6. Serve and enjoy.

Note: *Tuna is rich in zinc, selenium, vitamin C, and manganese. All these minerals work effectively in making our immune system strong. They are actually antioxidants that protect human bodies from various mishaps like cancer. They help in maintaining balance in the blood vessels, which, in turn, reduces the bad cholesterol in the human body. This fish is usually preferred by many people nowadays because of its property of being low in calories. This fish tastes great, which also provides its helping hand in meeting the daily requirement of nutrients as it is rich in nutrients and proteins with an essentially low amount of fat.*

Chicken Salad

Total Prep Time: 15 minutes
Yields: Two bowls
Nutrition Facts: Calories: 254 | Carbs: 3.3g | Protein: 19g | Fat: 18g | Fiber: 0.4g

Ingredients:

- One can of chicken or salmon or tuna. (They must be pre-cooked and make sure to get them after checking the ingredients as only seafood or meat, salt, and water are preferred.)
- One-eighth or one-fourth cup of olive or avocado oil
- Pinch of salt for taste
- Half an avocado
- One and a half teaspoon of lime juice

Method:

1. You will require a blender to prepare this. Scratch out the flesh from the avocado and place this flesh in the bowl of the blender. Along with it, add some juice from the lime, oil, and salt—process to form a creamy mixture.
2. Mix this creamy paste with tuna, salmon, or chicken (whatever you will prefer). Coat them properly.
3. On the serving plate, prepare a bed of the salad greens, and you may add some sweet potatoes or plantain or cassava chips to this bed.

Transfer the coated chicken or salmon or tuna over this bed of greens and enjoy.

Chapter 4: Dinner Recipes

Coconut Shrimp Soup

Total Prep & Cooking Time: 30 minutes
Yields: 4 servings
Nutrition Facts: Calories: 123.6 | Carbs: 2.7G |Protein: 12.4g | Fat: 6.4g | Fiber: 0g

Ingredients:

- One lime (quartered)
- One-fourth cup fresh cilantro (chopped)
- Six ounces of baby spinach
- One cup of diced one medium-sized tomato
- Half cup shredded cabbage
- Twelve ounces of medium-large sized shrimp (deveined and peeled)
- One cup (approximately four ounces) of sliced mushrooms
- One can of coconut milk (light)
- Two cups of chicken broth
- Two tbsps of Thai curry paste
- Two tsps coconut oil

Method:

1. At first, you have to take a large saucepan, pour oil, and heat it. Turn on the heat over medium-high.

2. Then you have to pour the curry paste and stir it. Sauté this for thirty seconds
3. Then add approximately half a cup of broth and start whisking together.
4. Then add the mushrooms, coconut milk, and the remaining broth. Simmer it for about ten minutes
5. Then add cabbage and shrimp. Reduce the heat to low and then cook for about five minutes.
6. Add tomatoes and spinach and then cook for about two more minutes.
7. Sprinkle cilantro and lime wedge and then serve.

Honey Lemon Chicken

Total Prep & Cooking Time: 21 minutes
Yields: 4 servings
Nutrition Facts: Calories: 265.1 | Carbs: 25.3G |
Protein: 31.1G | Fat: 7g | Fiber: 2.8g

Ingredients:

For meal prep,
- One head of broccoli
- Two divided lemons
- Three tablespoons of olive oil
- Half teaspoon salt
- Two large chicken breasts (or you can also take four to six boneless thighs)

For the sauce,
- One tablespoon olive oil
- Two tablespoons honey
- One teaspoon of dried oregano
- One-fourth cup of lemon juice (approximately one and a half lemons)

Method:

1. Start by cutting the chicken into small pieces. Toss them with half teaspoon salt.
2. Take a large skillet, turn the heat to medium, and then pour two tablespoons of olive oil. Heat it.

3. Cut a lemon into two halves. Take one part and remove its seeds.
4. Then add the lemon slices and the chicken pieces to the hot oil. You need to cook them for about four minutes before you flip them over.
5. While the chicken is cooking, start cutting down the broccoli and make florets. Whisk the florets together with the sauce.
6. Then flip the chicken on the other side and allow them to cook for about four more minutes.
7. Add sauce and broccoli florets mixture to the chicken and then reduce the heat to low.
8. Simmer for approximately five more minutes and then stir well so that the chicken gets fully coated with the sauce.

Are you enjoying this book? If so, i'd be really happy if you could leave a short review on Amazon, it means a lot to me! Thank you.

Chicken Pot Pie Soup

Total Prep & Cooking Time: 25 minutes
Yields: 4 servings
Nutrition Facts: Calories: 545 | Carbs: 40g | Protein: 22G | Fat: 35g | Fiber: 6g

Ingredients:

- Freshly chopped parsley leaves
- Black pepper (freshly chopped)
- One and a half teaspoons of dried sage
- One and a half teaspoons of salt
- Two tablespoons fresh thyme leaves
- One cup of cashews
- One cup of canned coconut cream or you can also use milk
- Two cups of chicken broth
- One pound of diced red potatoes
- Five to six minced garlic cloves
- Three sliced celery stalks
- Three diced carrots
- One diced onion
- Two tablespoons of olive oil or ghee
- Two large chicken breasts (skinless and boneless) chopped into small pieces

Method:

If you have an instant pot,

1. Take the instant pot and turn on the saute mode. Pour ghee. When the ghee is melted, add celery, carrots, and onion followed by regular stirring. Cook for some time, and when the onions become soft, add garlic. Continue to cook and stir continuously for about thirty seconds to one minute until a nice fragrance come out of it.
2. Add fresh thyme, dried sage, chicken, chicken broth, and potatoes to the instant pot. Secure the lid while the valve is in the sealing position. Cook them in manual high pressure for about ten minutes.
3. On the other hand, take a high-speed blender and add cashews and coconut milk. Blend until it becomes very smooth.
4. Then add the coconut-cashew mixture to the instant pot and season with salt and black pepper.

In case you don't have an instant pot, you can either do it in the slow cooker or on the stovetop.

In the slow cooker,

1. Over medium heat, take a large saucepan, add olive oil or ghee and then heat it. Sauté the celery, carrots, and onions until the onion gets softened. Then sauté the garlic for about one minute until a nice fragrance comes out. In your pot, transfer the sautéed mixture. Then

add Thyme, sage, chicken, chicken broth, and the potatoes to the pot.
2. Cover your pot and cook for about six hours on low heat or for about four hours on high heat.
3. Meanwhile, make the cashew coconut mixture, as stated above.
4. When the potatoes have become tender, pour the cashew-coconut mixture in and stir. Season it with salt and pepper.

On the stovetop,

1. On medium heat, take a large saucepan and heat the olive oil or ghee. Sauté the celery, carrots, and onions until the onion gets softened. Then sauté the garlic for about one minute until a nice fragrance comes out. In your pot, transfer the sautéed mixture. Then add Thyme, sage, chicken, chicken broth, and the potatoes to the pot.
2. Bring it to a boil and then cook for about four minutes.
3. Add the chicken breasts. Then cook for about six minutes until the potatoes become tender, and the chicken is nicely cooked.
4. Meanwhile, prepare the cashew-coconut mixture, as stated above.
5. To the pot, add the cashew coconut mixture and stir. Garnish with plenty of freshly cracked black pepper and salt.

Beef Goulash

Total Prep & Cooking Time: 1 hour 15 minutes
Yields: 4 servings
Nutrition Facts: Calories: 452 | Carbs: 7g | Protein:
20g | Fat: 38g | Fiber: 1G

Ingredients:

- One tbsp arrowroot powder (this is completely optional)
- Two tbsps (approx. 2G) fresh parsley
- One cup (approx 240ml) bone broth
- One tsp (approx. 2G) turmeric
- Two (approx. 100g) diced carrots
- Ten quartered white button mushrooms
- 450g of diced beef roast
- Four chopped and peeled garlic cloves
- One chopped and peeled medium-sized onion
- Four tbsps (approx. 60ml) avocado oil
- Salt

Method:

1. Take a pan, pour some olive oil, and heat it. Then add garlic and onions. Cook until they get softened. Then add the beef pieces and cook them until they are brown and slightly caramelized. Then add the carrots and mushrooms and then cook for about three to five minutes.

2. Add the beef broth and then reduce the heat to low. Cover the pan partially with a lid and then gently simmer for about one hour, paired with occasional stirring. You may need to add some water so that the mixture catching can be avoided.
3. You need to cook until the meat becomes tender and the sauce becomes consistent. In case it didn't get thickened enough, then remove the lid and try increasing the heat slowly until it gets thickened sufficiently.
4. Then you can add some arrowroot powder for thickening the sauce. Add salt as per your taste.
5. You can either serve it over mashed cauliflower or cauliflower rice. You can then try garnishing with freshly chopped parsley.

Chicken Alfredo

Total Prep & Cooking Time: 30 minutes
Yields: 2 servings
Nutrition Facts: Calories: 280 | Carbs: 31G | Protein: 16g | Fat: 0g | Fiber: 1G

Ingredients:

For preparing the sauce,
- Half tsp salt
- One tsp garlic powder
- One tsp dried basil
- Two tsps yeast
- One cup of coconut milk
- One and a half tbsps of arrowroot flour
- One cup of chicken broth

For meal prep,
- Salt
- Three-fourth pound of skinless and boneless chicken breasts
- Two tbsps coconut oil
- One pound zucchini

For garnishing,
- Freshly minced parsley

Method:

1. Cut the bottom portion and the top portion of the zucchini and cut in half. Use a spiralizer for making noodles from the zucchini.
2. Pat the chicken breast dry using a paper tunnel and then season it with salts on both sides. Take a skillet over medium heat, pour coconut oil and heat it. Add the chicken and cook for about eight minutes on each side until it turns golden and the inside is no longer pink. Take the chicken on a cutting board. Leave it for three minutes and then cut it into strips (approx. half-inch thick).
3. Then take a bowl, add arrowroot flour and chicken broth and whisk until the flour gets nicely dissolved to avoid lumps (you can also use a blender).
4. In the same skillet, add garlic, basil, yeast, coconut milk, and salt and whisk together. Boil it over medium heat. Reduce the heat to medium-low and then add the chicken broth mixture. Stir constantly for about two minutes until the sauce gets thickened. Season it as per your taste.
5. In the skillet, add the zucchini noodles and toss. Check whether the noodles are completely coated with the sauce or not. Take the noodles on a plate, top it with chicken slices, and garnish them with freshly minced parsley. Serve!

Tuscan Chicken Soup

Total Prep & Cooking Time: 1 hour
Yields: 4 servings
Nutrition Facts: Calories: 412 | Carbs: 52G | Protein:
31G | Fat: 9g | Fiber: 9g

Ingredients:

- Two tablespoons of parmesan (finely grated)
- Freshly chopped parsley
- 100g of chopped kale
- Two skinless chicken breasts (cooked and shredded)
- 400g of cooked cannellini beans (nicely washed and drained)
- Half teaspoon black pepper
- Half teaspoon salt
- One liter of chicken stock
- Two peeled and diced medium-sized potatoes
- Two peeled and chopped medium-sized carrots
- One sliced celery stick
- Half tsp dried thyme two fresh thyme sprigs
- Two peeled and minced garlic cloves
- One peeled and chopped onion
- One tablespoon olive oil
- Granary bread, toasted (for serving)
- Fresh thyme

Method:

1. Take a large saucepan and heat the oil. Add onions, turn the heat on medium-low and cook for about ten minutes paired with constant stirring until it becomes soft.
2. Add the thyme and garlic and cook for about two more minutes. Add the potatoes, carrots, and celery and stir. Then add the chicken broth, pepper, and salt.
3. Take the drained cannellini beans and add them to the saucepan and cook for five more minutes.
4. Then you have to add the shredded chicken and heat for two to three minutes. Add kale. Start Stirring and simmer for about one to two minutes until the kale is withered. Season it with salt and pepper as per your taste.
5. Divide it into four bowls, and then garnish it with a few thyme sprigs, grated parmesan, and freshly chopped parsley. Serve it with toasted granary bread.

Chicken Kofta Curry

Total Prep & Cooking Time: 45 minutes
Yields: 4 servings
Nutrition Facts: Calories: 229 | Carbs: 9g | Protein: 25G | Fat: 9g | Fiber: 2G

Ingredients:

For preparing the chicken meatballs,
- One teaspoon oil
- One teaspoon red chili powder
- One-eighth teaspoon turmeric
- Handful of cilantro
- One green chili (small)
- Three cloves of garlic
- Half inch ginger
- Two tablespoons of wheat flour (or you can also use rice flour)
- One pound of ground chicken
- Salt to taste

For preparing the gravy,
- One tablespoon oil
- One-eighth teaspoon turmeric
- One teaspoon garam masala
- One tablespoon red chili powder
- Three pureed tomatoes
- Three cloves of garlic
- One-fourth inch of ginger
- Two tablespoons of grated coconut

- One thinly sliced medium-sized onion
- Cilantro (for garnishing)
- Salt to taste

Method:

1. Turn the heat on medium-low. Place a heavy bottom pan on it and roast the grated coconut for about two minutes. Then keep aside the coconut. In the same pan, pour some oil, add the sliced onions and saute on medium-low heat for about twenty minutes until the onions turn golden brown.
2. Meanwhile, take a handful of cilantro, green chili, garlic, and ginger and make a fine paste. Mix it with salt, wheat flour, red chili powder, turmeric, and minced chicken. Take some oil in your hands and make small balls from this mixture and keep them aside.
3. Take out the browned onions from the pan. Take cilantro, garlic, ginger, browned onions, and roasted coconuts and make a paste.
4. In the same pan, heat some oil and add the pureed tomatoes and the masala paste to it— Cook for about five to seven minutes on medium heat. Then add turmeric, garam masala, and red chili powder. Add salt and mix well. Then add a three-fourth cup of water and again mix. After the gravy comes to a boil, place the keema balls on top of the gravy. Cover the pan and cook for another ten minutes on medium-low heat.

5. Stir and cook for five more minutes. You can garnish it with freshly chopped cilantro.
6. You can serve it with thin rice flour crepes or steamed basmati rice.

Fennel and Spinach Soup

Total Prep & Cooking Time: 35 minutes
Yields: 8 servings
Nutrition Facts: Calories: 96 | Carbs: 13G | Protein: 4g
| Fat: 3.8g | Fiber: 3g

Ingredients:

- One tsp lemon juice
- One tsp of grated lemon rind
- Half cup yogurt
- One-fourth tsp of black pepper (freshly ground)
- Four ounces of spinach
- One bay leaf
- One cup of water
- Two cups of chicken broth (low sodium content and fat-free)
- Three-eighth tsp salt
- One tbsp freshly chopped thyme
- One cup of chopped shallots
- Two cups of chopped leek
- Two tbsps of extra-virgin olive oil
- Two big fennel bulbs (stalks present)
- Two red bell peppers
- Grounded red pepper

Method:

1. Preheat the broiler. Cut down the bell peppers lengthwise in halves (discard the membrane and seed). Take a foil-lined baking sheet and place the pepper halves (skin sides up and flattened with hand). Broil for about fifteen minutes until blackened. Place it in a paper bag and fold for closing tightly. Peel it and then chop it and then set aside.
2. Then you need to trim the tough outer leaves from the fennel. The feather fronds (to measure two tablespoons) need to be minced and kept aside. Stalks need to be removed and discarded. Cut the bulbs lengthwise in halves. Chop them to measure about four cups.
3. Heat some oil over medium heat. Add leek, fennel bulbs, salt, and other ingredients. Cover it and cook for about ten minutes. Stir occasionally. Add bay leaf, water, and broth and bring them to a boil. Cover it and lower the heat. Simmer for about twelve minutes. Discard the bay leaves. Put the black pepper and spinach and stir. Take it down from the heat, cover it, and leave it for about five minutes at room temperature.
4. Pour half of the fennel mixture in a blender. From the blender lid, remove the centerpiece to allow the steam to escape. Then secure the blender lid. Blend it until it becomes smooth. Then pour it into a large bowl. Repeat the exact same procedure for the remaining fennel mixture. Again take the pureed soup to the pan

and heat it over medium heat for two more minutes until it is thoroughly heated.

5. Then in a food processor, combine ground red pepper, lemon juice, lemon rind, yogurt, and roasted bell peppers. Process until it becomes smooth.

6. On each soup bowl, add two tablespoons of yogurt mixture and garnish with the fennel fronds. Serve!

Shepherd's Pie

Total Prep & Cooking Time: 1 hour 15 minutes
Yields: 8 servings
Nutrition Facts: Calories: 407 | Carbs: 26g | Protein: 21G | Fat: 24g | Fiber: 3g

Ingredients:

For preparing the beef mixture,
- One teaspoon of freshly minced rosemary
- One teaspoon of freshly minced thyme
- Two and a half tablespoons of tomato paste
- Three-fourth cup of beef bone broth (or you can also use chicken bone broth)
- Pinch of salt for the veggies
- Two minced garlic cloves
- One chopped medium-sized onion
- One and a half cup of chopped Brussels sprouts
- One cup of diced carrots
- Pepper and salt (for the seasoning of the beef)
- One and a half pounds of ground beef
- One tablespoon ghee

For the mashed potatoes,
- Freshly chopped parsley
- Salt and pepper
- Three tablespoons of yeast
- Three tablespoons ghee
- Two-third cup of coconut milk (nicely blended before adding)

- Four to six russet potatoes (cut into pieces each of two inches size)

Method:

For preparing the potatoes,

1. Take a three-quarter pot with water and heat it. Sprinkle some salt and then bring it to a boil. Add the potato pieces (two inches each) into the boiling water. Cook it until it becomes soft.
2. Strain out the water and keep the potatoes in the pot. Then in the same pot, add coconut milk and ghee. Turn the heat on low and then mash the potatoes using a potato masher. Turn off the heat when it becomes smooth and then add yeast, pepper, and salt. After this, you can use an immersion blender if you want a creamy texture for your potatoes.

For preparing the beef mixture and baking pie,

1. At first, preheat your oven to three hundred and seventy-five degrees.
2. Take an ovenproof skillet, add beef, and sprinkle some salt. Turn the heat on medium-high and cook the beef until brown and break lumps with a spoon. Then on a plate, put the beef with a slotted spoon. Then keep it aside.
3. Turn the heat to medium and then add carrot and Brussels sprouts to the skillet. Then stir for coating and then cook for about two minutes.

Add onions and cook until it gets soft. Sprinkle veggies with some salt, add garlic and stir. Then you have to cover the skillet so that the carrot gets soft and tender.

4. Add the rest of the ingredients, in the skillet, for the beef mixture. Stir for combining. Then place the beef in the skillet. Keep stirring for coating the beef fully and then simmer for about two minutes until the sauce gets thickened, and the flavors blend in.

5. Over the beef mixture, spread the mashed potatoes. You can use a spatula or a spoon for smoothening the top. Sprinkle some parsley. Then on a large baking sheet, place the skillet and then bake it in the oven (which is already preheated) for approximately twenty minutes. Bake until u see the top is beginning to turn light brown, and the sauce is bubbling.

6. Take out the skillet from the oven and leave it for about ten minutes. Then serve it hot!

Chicken Cacciatore

Total Prep & Cooking Time: 50 minutes
Yields: 6 servings
Nutrition Facts: Calories: 346 | Carbs: 17G | Protein:
23G | Fat: 22G | Fiber: 4g

Ingredients:

- Fresh parsley
- One-third cup of pitted olives
- Red pepper (crushed)
- Salt and black pepper
- One teaspoon dried thyme
- One teaspoon of dried oregano
- One to two tablespoons of tomato paste
- Twenty-eight ounces of crushed tomatoes (basil present)
- One-third cup of chicken bone broth
- One diced red bell pepper
- Eight ounces of sliced white mushrooms
- Two diced large carrots
- Four minced garlic cloves
- One diced small onion
- One to two tablespoons of olive oil (you can also use avocado oil)
- Black pepper and salt
- Six chicken thighs (skin on, with bone)

Method:

1. Season the chicken on both sides using pepper and salt.
2. Take a large, heavy skillet, pour some oil, and heat it over medium-high heat. Place the chicken and sear each side for about five minutes until it turns deep golden brown. Remove it from the skillet and place it on a plate and keep it aside. Keep the remaining fat in the skillet intact.
3. Reduce the heat to medium and then cook the onions for about one to two minutes until it becomes fragrant and translucent. Then add the garlic and sauté it for about thirty seconds until a nice fragrance comes out of it.
4. Add the mushrooms, carrot, and peppers and sauté it for about five minutes until the vegetables become soft.
5. Push the veggies aside, and again add the chicken to the skillet. Then pour in the broth, tomato paste, and crushed tomatoes. Season it with crushed red pepper, thyme, oregano, black pepper, and salt.
6. Mix the sauce, keep it uncovered, and simmer it for about five minutes. Then you have to cover and turn the heat on medium-low and simmer it for about twenty-five to thirty-five minutes paired with occasional stirring until the chicken is nicely cooked. Put olives and stir, and garnish with freshly chopped parsley or some other herb as per your choice.

7. You can serve it with roasted veggies. You can
    also serve it over cauliflower rice or zucchini
    noodles to keep it low carb.

Lemon Parsley Swordfish

Total Prep & Cooking Time: 25 minutes
Yields: 4 servings
Nutrition Facts: Calories: 390 | Carbs: 1G | Protein: 37g | Fat: 26g | Fiber: 0g

Ingredients:

- One-fourth tsp of red pepper flakes (crushed)
- Two tsps of minced garlic
- One tbsp lemon juice
- One-third cup of olive oil
- Half cup freshly minced parsley
- Half tsp salt
- Four swordfish steaks (each weighing seven ounces)

Method:

1. At first, you need to preheat your oven to four hundred and twenty-five degrees. Take a nicely greased baking dish and place the fish and then sprinkle some salt. Then take a bowl and combine pepper flakes, garlic, lemon juice, oil, and one-fourth cup parsley. Spoon this mixture over the fish.
2. You need to keep the fish uncovered and bake it for about fifteen to twenty minutes until the fish gets flaked easily by a fork. Keep it moist by basting it occasionally and sprinkle the rest of the parsley on top of it.

**Honey Ginger Shrimp Bowls**

Total Prep & Cooking Time: 26 minutes
Yields: 2 servings
Nutrition Facts: Calories: 165.9 | Carbs: 4.1G | Protein: 19g | Fat: 8.1G | Fiber: 0.8g

Ingredients:

For preparing the shrimp,
- Freshly ground pepper, salt, and lime
- Two teaspoons of avocado oil
- Two minced garlic cloves
- One teaspoon minced ginger
- Two tablespoons of coconut aminos
- Two tablespoons of honey
- Twelve ounces of uncooked shrimp (deveined and peeled)

For preparing the salad,
- One sliced avocado
- One-fourth cilantro (chopped)
- Four sliced green onions
- Half cup radishes (shredded)
- Half cup carrots (shredded)
- Four cups spinach (or any greens as per your choice, preferably spinach and arugula)

For the dressing,
- Salt and pepper
- One-fourth teaspoon of ginger powder

- One-fourth teaspoon of garlic powder
- One teaspoon honey
- One teaspoon coconut aminos
- Two tablespoons of olive oil
- Two tablespoons of lime juice

Method:

1. At first, you have to take a bowl and combine ginger, garlic, coconut aminos, and honey. Start whisking.
2. Then you'll need to take a lidded container and place the shrimp. Then take the prepared marinade and pour over the shrimp and stir.
3. Then you need to leave this in the refrigerator to marinate for two hours. Meanwhile, you have to start preparing the dressing and also the salad.
4. Take a skillet, turn the heat to medium-high, and heat the avocado oil. Then pour the marinade and the shrimp into it. The shrimp needs to be cooked on one side, for about three minutes, until it turns opaque (when the shrimp will be fully cooked, you can see a pink exterior and a soft white inner flesh). Then flip onto the other side and cook for three more minutes. The shrimp needs to get fully cooked (try not to overcook), and the sauce needs to get thickened enough for coating the shrimp. Then start seasoning the shrimp with lime juice, salt, and pepper.

5. Then you need to take a large bowl and toss the radishes, carrots, and salad greens. Then you'll have to divide the mixture into two different plates.
6. Then top the salad mixture with avocado, lime wedges, cilantro, green onions, and shrimp.
7. Then do the dressing with lime juice, coconut aminos, honey, garlic powder, ginger powder, salt, and pepper. Serve!

Thai Chicken Soup

Total Prep & Cooking Time: 4 hours 10 minutes
Yields: 4 servings
Nutrition Facts: Calories: 185 | Carbs: 5g | Protein: 13g | Fat: 14g | Fiber: 0.7g

Ingredients:

- Three inches piece of lemongrass
- One teaspoon of ground ginger
- One tablespoon honey
- One to two cups of chicken broth
- One tablespoon of fish sauce
- One tablespoon of coconut aminos
- One tablespoon of lime juice
- Two tablespoons of minced garlic
- One diced small yellow onion or shallot.
- Two pounds of skinless and boneless chicken thighs, which is cut into small (one inch) pieces.
- Ingredients needed only while cooking: half cup chopped cilantro, half cup chopped basil, three green onions (sliced), coconut milk.

Method:

For stovetop,

1. Take a large saucepan, then put all the contents of the bag into it. Then add coconut milk.

2. Bring it to a boil. Then reduce the heat and then simmer for about seven to nine minutes.
3. Cook until the chicken gets nicely cooked.
4. Then garnish with cilantro, basil, and green onions.

For slow cooker,

1. In a slow cooker, put all the contents of the bag.
2. Add coconut milk and then on low heat, cook for about two to four hours.
3. Then garnish with cilantro, basil, and green onions.

Chapter 5: Snack Recipes

Banana Bread Protein Balls

Total Prep & Cooking Time: Thirteen minutes
Yields: Eight balls
Nutrition Facts: Calories: 183 | Carbs: 18g | Protein: 4g | Fat: 10g | Fiber: 2G

Ingredients:

- Half a cup of vanilla or neutral protein powder
- One-fourth of a cup each of
- Coconut flour
- Shredded coconut
- Toasted coconut butter (or, sub-almond butter for non-AIP recipes)
- Ripe bananas, mashed
- Half a teaspoon of Ceylon cinnamon

Method:

1. Add all the ingredients in a food processor and mix them well.
2. When they have combined properly, and the dough has formed, take the dough out of the processor and roll it into balls.
3. Take a parchment paper-lined Tupperware or plate and keep the balls on it.
4. Store them in the refrigerator until ready to eat.

Note: *Collagen protein is recommended if you want a truly AIP compliant protein powder. Do not use peanut butter for this recipe because peanut butter is too oily.*

Baked Plantains

Total Prep & Cooking Time: Twenty-five minutes
Yields: Six servings
Nutrition Facts: Calories: 173 | Carbs: 28g | Protein: 1G | Fat: 7g | Fiber: 2G

Ingredients:

- Three tablespoons of olive oil (or coconut oil)
- Three ripe plantains (dark yellow in color with black spots)
- One teaspoon of salt

Method:

1. Preheat your oven to 425 degrees Fahrenheit.
2. Take a baking sheet and line it with parchment paper.
3. Remove the ends of each of the three plantains. Score the peels from one end to the other while making sure that you don't cut through the plantain. Remove the peels by pulling them off.
4. Cut the plantains into quarter-inch to one-third inch thick pieces. Cut at an angle to make longer pieces.
5. Place the slices of plantain on the baking sheet and drizzle some oil on them. Toss to coat oil on both the sides of the plantain strips. Place them in a single layer and generously sprinkle salt on them.

6. Keep the baking sheets in the oven and let it bake for ten minutes. Then take it out and flip the plantain strips and allow it to bake for another ten minutes. Baking the plantains at high heat will make your plantains crispy around the edges before they absorb all the oil.
7. Serve them immediately or at room temperature.
8. You can make these baked plantains ahead of time and store them in airtight containers for up to one week in the refrigerator. You can easily reheat them by placing them in the oven for a few minutes at 350 degrees Fahrenheit so that they get slightly hot.

Note: You can add nutmeg or cinnamon powder if you want to spice up your plantains. You can sprinkle garlic powder, cayenne pepper, and cumin on the plantains if you want a spicy-hot version.

Coconut Turmeric Snack Balls

Total Prep & Cooking Time: Ten minutes
Yields: Four servings
Nutrition Facts: Calories: 413 | Carbs: 23G | Protein: 4g | Fat: 35g | Fiber: 9g

Ingredients:

- Three tablespoons (or forty-five ml) of raw honey
- One tablespoon (or six grams) of turmeric powder
- Half a cup (or 120 ml) or coconut butter
- One and a quarter of a cup (or hundred grams) of shredded coconut (unsweetened)

Method:

1. Slightly melt the honey and coconut butter together. Add the turmeric powder and unsweetened shredded coconut into the mixture and stir everything together.
2. Add the mixture into ice cube trays and keep it in the freezer for two hours.
3. Defrost the snack balls for about ten minutes before serving them.

Note: _The nutritional data mentioned above are estimates and based on per serving quantities._

Red Velvet Smoothie

Total Prep & Cooking Time: Ten minutes
Yields: One serving
Nutrition Facts: Calories: 105 | Carbs: 19g | Protein: 1G | Fat: 3g | Fiber: 3g

Ingredients:

- Half a cup each of
- Crushed ice
- Full-fat coconut milk (about 120 ml)
- One tablespoon each of
- Carob powder (about six grams)
- Coconut cream (about fifteen ml), to drizzle (optional)
- One banana (about a hundred grams), peeled and chopped into pieces
- One large beet (about ninety-eight grams), cooked, peeled, and chopped

Method:

1. Add the crushed ice, coconut milk, banana, and beets into a blender and blitz until you get a fairly smooth blend.
2. Pour the smoothie into a glass and add a drizzle of whisked coconut milk on top before serving.

**Note**: All the nutritional data mentioned above are estimates and based on per serving quantities.

Avocado Coconut Smoothie

Total Prep & Cooking Time: Five minutes
Yields: Two servings
Nutrition Facts: Calories: 265 | Carbs: 10g | Protein:
3g | Fat: 26g | Fiber: 7g

Ingredients:

- One teaspoon (about five ml) of raw honey, to taste
- Half a cup (about 120 ml) of unsweetened coconut milk, plus more if you have difficulty getting the mixture to blend
- One cup (about 240 gm.) of ice
- One avocado

Method:

1. Slice a ripe avocado in half.
2. Scoop out the flesh of the avocado with the help of a spoon.
3. Add the avocado flesh, raw honey, coconut milk, and ice into a blender and blend properly. Start slow and slowly increase the speed of the blender.
4. You can add more coconut milk if required and blend it until you get a smooth mixture.
5. Pour the smoothie into two glasses and serve cold.

Note*: The nutritional data mentioned above are estimates and based on per serving quantities.*

Blueberry Coconut Yogurt Smoothie

Total Prep & Cooking Time: Five minutes
Yields: Two servings
Nutrition Facts: Calories: 70 | Carbs: 2G | Protein: 2G |
Fat: 5g | Fiber: 0g

Ingredients:

- One cup of coconut milk
- Ten blueberries
- One pot of coconut yogurt (about 120 ml)

Method:

1. Add the blueberries, coconut milk, and coconut yogurt into a blender and blend properly until you get a smooth blend. The stevia, blueberries, as well as vanilla extract, add plenty of sweetness to this smoothie. You can add a dash of honey if you think you need more sweetness.
2. Pour the smoothie into two glasses and serve as a snack or a quick, nutritious breakfast smoothie.

**Note**: The nutritional data mentioned above are estimates and based on per serving quantities.

Lemon Fried Avocado

Total Prep & Cooking Time: 7 minutes
Yields: Two servings
Nutrition Facts: Calories: | Carbs: | Protein: | Fat: |
Fiber:

Ingredients:

- One tablespoon each of
- Lemon juice
- Coconut oil
- One ripe avocado, pieced into slices
- Salt or lemon to taste

Method:

1. Cut an avocado in half and remove the stone. Score the flesh inside to cut it into slices.
2. Heat a frying pan and add the coconut oil into it.
3. Gently place the slices of avocado in the oil and fry them. Turn them gently midway so that all the sides get browned.
4. Squeeze some lemon juice and sprinkle the salt on top of the slices.
5. Serve warm.

**Note**: The nutritional data mentioned above are estimates and based on per serving quantities.

Raspberry Tart

Total Prep & Cooking Time: Two hours and ten minutes
Yields: Eight servings
Nutrition Fact: Calories: 263 | Carbs: 20g | Protein: 8g | Fat: 18g | Fiber: 9g

Ingredients:

For the pie crust,
- One-fourth of a cup each of
- Water (about sixty ml)
- Coconut flour (about twenty-eight grams)
- Ground flaxseed (about twenty-eight grams)
- One cup of almond flour (about 120 grams)

For soaking the cashews,
- One cup of cashews, unsalted and unroasted (about 150 grams)

For the cashew layer,
- Two tablespoons each of
- Hot water (about 30 ml)
- Erythritol (about 24 grams)
- One tablespoon of powdered gelatin (about six grams)
- Five and a half tablespoons of unsweetened almond milk (about 80 ml)
- One teaspoon of vanilla extract (about 5 ml)

- Reserved soaking cashew nuts

For finishing the tart,
- Powdered Erythritol (for dusting)
- Forty to fifty raspberries

Method:

1. Keep the cashew nuts in a bowl and cover it completely with hot filtered water. Cover the bowl with a dish towel or a cling film and allow the cashews to soak overnight.
2. Make the pie crust on the following day. Preheat your oven to 175 degrees Celsius or 350 degrees Fahrenheit.
3. Combine the almond flour, coconut flour, ground flaxseed with a quarter cup of water and make a dough. Grease a tart or pie pan and press the dough into it. Without wheat flour, the tart crust depends on the perfect blend of flax meal, coconut flour, and almond flour for the perfect tender crust, which will form the base of the dessert. As almond flour has a high content of fat, additional fat can be skipped in favor of water, which acts as a binder.
4. Keep the pie or tart pan in the oven and let it bake for ten to twelve minutes so that the crust gets slightly browned.
5. After the crust turns brown, take the tart pan out of the oven and keep it aside to cool.
6. Drain the cashews in the meantime and reserve one-third cup of the soaking water. Add the

drained cashews and one-third cup of the reserved water in a blender or food processor and mix them properly. Don't forget to pause and regularly scrape down the sides of the bowl.

7. Add the Erythritol and almond milk into the blender or food processor and keep mixing them together until you get a smooth mixture.

8. To make the gelatin egg, take a small bowl with about one tablespoon (about fifteen ml) of lukewarm water and sprinkle the powdered gelatin over it. When the gelatin dissolves, mix in one tablespoon (about fifteen ml) of very hot water until it dissolves completely.

9. Add this hot gelatin mixture into the blender or food processor containing the creamy cashew mixture and blend properly to combine them together.

10. Add the creamy cashew mixture into the cooled tart crust. Keep it in the refrigerator for at least two hours until it gets set.

11. Arrange the raspberries on top of the tart filling before serving the tart and dust the powdered Erythritol on top of it for a perfect finish.

12. You can keep any leftover tart in the refrigerator and eat it later.

Note: The nutritional data mentioned above are estimates and based on per serving quantities.

Zucchini Fries

Total Prep & Cooking Time: Twenty-five minutes
Yields: Six servings
Nutrition Facts: Calories: 90 | Carbs: 12G | Protein: 4g
| Fat: 2G | Fiber: 4g

Ingredients:

- One cup (about 112 grams) of coconut flour
- Five zucchinis (about six hundred grams)
- Two teaspoons (about nine grams) of salt
- Two tablespoons (about fourteen grams) of onion powder

Method:

1. Preheat your oven to 200 degrees Celsius or 390 degrees Fahrenheit.
2. Slice the zucchini in half and eliminate the inner fleshy region. Dice the sliced zucchinis into quarter-inch fries. Try cutting the zucchinis into fairly skinny strips for crispy, crunchy fries. As zucchinis are quite moist, you can dry them out with a paper towel after cutting them into pieces.
3. Add the coconut flour, onion powder, and salt in a bowl and mix them together and then add in the slices of zucchini and toss them to coat.
4. Take a baking dish and grease it. Place the zucchini slices evenly on the greased baking sheet.

5. Keep it in the oven and allow it to bake for about twenty to thirty minutes. Pause halfway and turn them over. Remember to give the fries enough time in the oven. Otherwise, taking them out too quickly might leave the fries sad and limp. When the fries get golden and crispy around the edges, take them out of the oven.
6. Serve immediately as these zucchini fries are best enjoyed straight out of the oven. If you try to keep them for another day, they might get floppy and mushy.

Note*: The nutritional data mentioned above are estimates and based on per serving quantities.*

Carrot Gummies

Total Prep & Cooking Time: Two hours and ten
minutes
Yields: Six servings
Nutrition Facts: Calories: 36 | Carbs: 4g | Protein: 5g |
Fat: 0g | Fiber: 0g

Ingredients:

- Five tablespoons of gelatin powder (about
  thirty-five grams)
- Two cups of carrot juice plus some of the pulp
  (about 480 ml)

Method:

1. Place a small pot on the stove and add the
   carrot juice into it.
2. Heat the carrot juice on medium heat until the
   liquid begins to simmer.
3. Add a small amount of gelatin and at a time
   and stir it in until it's completely dissolved.
4. Strain the liquid with the help of a strainer to
   eliminate any lumps that might have formed.
5. Pour the strained liquid equally into silicone
   molds or ice cube trays. You can also use candy
   molds and create any shape that you want.
   Then, keep them in the refrigerator for at least
   two hours so that they set to form gummies.

Note: *The nutritional data mentioned above are estimates and based on per serving quantities.*

Nori Bites

Total Prep & Cooking Time: Fifteen minutes
Yields: Eight bites
Nutrition Facts: Calories: 152 | Carbs: 3g | Protein: 15G | Fat: 7g | Fiber: 1G

Ingredients:

For the nori bites,
- One-fourth of a carrot (about thirteen grams), peeled and cut into matchsticks
- One-fourth of a cucumber (about fifty-five grams), sliced into thin sticks
- One green onion (about five grams), sliced
- ounces of smoked salmon (about 148 grams)
- Two nori sheets
- Cilantro, for garnishing

For the sauce,
- One teaspoon of coconut aminos (about five ml)
- Three tablespoons of coconut cream (about 45 ml)

Method:

1. To make the sauce, simply mix the coconut aminos and the coconut cream properly and then set it aside.

2. Slice the nori sheets into four equal pieces so that you can create eight tiny squares with them. Run a damp finger over the sheets and dampen them slightly until you can easily roll them up.
3. Add a small amount of the sauce on top of each square. Then add the carrots, cucumber, green onion, and smoked salmon onto each piece.
4. Roll up the squares, and your nori bites are ready to be served. You can add some cilantro on top as a garnish.

Note: *The nutritional data mentioned above are estimates and based on per serving quantities.*

**Ambrosia Berry Salad**

Total Prep & Cooking Time: Five minutes
Yields: Four servings
Nutrition Facts: Calories: 187 | Carbs: 16g | Protein: 0g | Fat: 14g | Fiber: 5g

Ingredients:

- Three and a half ounces (about hundred grams) each of
- Fresh pineapple, chopped into small pieces
- Fresh raspberries
- Fresh blackberries
- Fresh blueberries
- One cup (about 240 ml) of coconut cream (or taken from the top of a can of coconut milk kept in the refrigerator)
- Two tablespoons of shredded coconut (about ten grams), for garnishing (optional)

Method:

1. Using a handheld mixer or a whisk, whip the coconut cream so that it gets slightly thickened.
2. In a bowl, add the chopped pineapple and berries and stir them gently with a rubber spatula to combine them with the thickened coconut cream.
3. Pour the ambrosia salad equally into four bowls.

4. Before serving, you can add the shredded coconut as a garnish if you want.

Note: *The nutritional data mentioned above are estimates and based on per serving quantities.*

**Raspberry Ripple Ice Cream**

Total Prep & Cooking Time: Thirty minutes plus freeze time
Yields: Six servings
Nutrition Facts: Calories: 358 | Carbs: 34g | Protein: 2G | Fat: 25G | Fiber: 12G

Ingredients:

- One-fourth of a cup of honey (about sixty ml)
- Two cans (each of 400 ml) of coconut milk (full-fat) kept at room temperature
- Six ounces of fresh raspberries (about 170 grams)

Method:

1. Add the raspberries into a food processor or blender and blend it until you get a smooth puree. Keep it aside.
2. Shake the cans of coconut milk that are kept at room temperature and pour it into a large bowl. Whisk the coconut milk properly to remove all the lumps.
3. Add the honey into the bowl containing coconut milk and whisk to combine them together.
4. Pour this mixture of coconut cream and honey into an ice-cream maker and churn as per the instructions provided by the manufacturer.

5. Add this churned ice-cream into a freezer-safe container that can be closed. Fold in the raspberry puree gently into the ice cream and create a swirl pattern.
6. Close the lid of the container and keep the raspberry ice cream in the freezer to set.
7. You can store any leftover ice cream in the freezer to enjoy it later.

__Note__: The nutritional data mentioned above are estimates and based on per serving quantities.

Mixed Berry Crumble

Total Prep & Cooking Time: Twenty-five minutes
Yields: Six servings
Nutrition Facts: Calories: 436 | Carbs: 76g | Protein: 2G | Fat: 14g | Fiber: 32G

Ingredients:

- Three-fourth of a cup of shredded coconut (about sixty grams)
- Three tablespoons of solid coconut oil (about 54 grams)
- Six tablespoons of cassava flour (about 45 grams)
- Six and a half tablespoons of coconut flour (about 45 grams)
- One tablespoon of lemon juice (about 15 ml)
- Five cups of mixed berries (about 900 grams)
- Extra shredded coconut (optional)

Method:

1. Preheat your oven to 175 degrees Celsius or 350 degrees Fahrenheit.
2. Add all the mixed berries and the lemon juice into a bowl. Squish the berries gently and mix them properly with the lemon juice.
3. Divide this berry mixture equally between six oven-proof ramekins. Remember to place the ramekins on a tray beforehand. Bake them in the oven for about fifteen to twenty minutes.

4. In the meantime, mix the cassava flour and coconut flour together. Cut the solid coconut oil into tiny portions and add them into the flour mix. Rub the mixture with your hands until you get a coarse breadcrumb-like texture. Add in the shredded coconut to this mixture and stir everything together.
5. Remove the ramekin tray from the oven once the berries are baked and add the crumb mixture equally and evenly over the six ramekins.
6. Place the ramekins back in the oven and allow them to cook for five to eight extra minutes. Remove them from the oven when the tops turn golden and crispy.
7. For some extra crunch, add some more shredded coconut on the top as a garnish.

Note*: As the berries bake, the crumb mixture will melt and get absorbed by the berries. This is a good thing as this will thicken up the berry mixture. All the nutritional data mentioned above are estimates and based on per serving quantities.*

Sweet Potato Cookies

Total Prep & Cooking Time: 40 minutes
Yields: Eight servings
Nutrition Facts: Calories: 128 | Carbs: 15G | Protein:
3g | Fat: 6g | Fiber: 4g

Ingredients:

- Three-fourth of a cup of coconut flour (about 84 grams)
- Seven ounces of sweet potatoes (about 200 grams), peeled and grated
- One teaspoon of baking powder (about two grams)
- One-fourth of a cup of honey (about 60 ml)
- One tablespoon of powdered gelatin (about six grams)
- Three tablespoons of coconut oil (about 45 ml)

Method:

1. Preheat your oven to 175 degrees Celsius or 350 degrees Fahrenheit.
2. Place a pan over low heat and add the coconut oil into it. Then add the shredded sweet potatoes and cook over low heat. Stir them at regular intervals to release the moisture from the sweet potatoes and cook it out.
3. In the meantime, make a gelatin egg mixing the gelatin powder with one tablespoon (about fifteen ml) of lukewarm water. When the

gelatin dissolves, add a tablespoon (about fifteen ml) of boiling hot water into it and mix it properly until the gelatin gets dissolved completely. The gelatin eggs act like a binder similar to how the protein in egg whites work.

4. Add the honey into the sweet potatoes once they have softened and stir properly. Cook the potatoes until all the moisture has disappeared from it.
5. Pour the gelatin mixture into the sweet potato mixture and mix them properly.
6. Remove the pan from the stove and add in three-fourths of a cup along with two tablespoons of hot water (about 240ml). Keep this sweet potato mixture aside.
7. Take a large bowl and mix the coconut flour with the baking soda in it.
8. Add the sweet potato mixture into the bowl containing the flour mixture and combine them together with the help of a wooden spoon.
9. Divide the mixture into balls of about two and a half tablespoons (40 ml) size. Then flatten them into cookie shapes with your hands.
10. Line a baking tray with a parchment paper and place the cookies on them. Flatten the cookies again with the palm of your clean hands and make one-third of an inch or 1Cm high rough shapes. You can use a cookie cutter to press each shape. However, remember not to remove and discard any excess. Keep it on the tray.
11. Keep it in the preheated oven and let it bake for about twenty minutes.

12. Turn off the oven after twenty minutes with opening the door of the oven. Keep the cookies in the oven for another hour to let them cook in the residual heat.
13. Remove the tray from the oven when the cookies have cooled down a little and remove the extra cut-offs from the cookies.
14. Serve the cookies after they have cooled down completely.

Note: The nutritional data mentioned above are estimates and based on per serving quantities.

Pineapple Fruit Salsa

Total Prep & Cooking Time: Twenty minutes
Yields: Four servings
Nutrition Facts: Calories: 30.9 | Carbs: 7.4g| Protein:
0.4g | Fat: 0.4g | Fiber: 0.8g

Ingredients:

- One cup each of
- Blueberries
- Strawberries, diced
- One pineapple
- One-fourth of a cup of lemon juice, freshly squeezed
- Two kiwis, peeled and cut into pieces
- One teaspoon each of
- Coconut sugar
- Cinnamon

Method:

1. Cut the pineapple down the middle. Eliminate the core and hollow out the flesh.
2. Cut the pineapple into small pieces and place it in a large bowl. Add in the kiwis, blueberries, and strawberries and mix well.
3. Take a small ramekin and add the cinnamon, coconut sugar, and lemon juice. Combine them together. The freshly squeezed lemon juice enhances the taste and maintains the freshness of the fruits for a longer period of time, while

the warm cinnamon increases the naturally
sweet flavors of the fruit. Add this mixture over
the fruits and toss to combine everything
together.

4. Place the fruit salsa into the hollowed
    pineapple bowl and serve.

5. If you want to prepare the pineapple fruit salsa
    ahead of time, keep the lemon juice mixture
    and fruit separately to keep it fresh. Toss the
    lemon juice mixture with the fruit salsa when
    you're ready to serve and then add it into the
    pineapple bowl.

Bacon-Wrapped Avocado Fries

Total Prep & Cooking Time: Forty minutes
Yields: Twenty servings
Nutrition Facts: Calories: 65 | Carbs: 0.8g | Protein:
4g | Fat: 5.1G | Fiber: 0.5g

Ingredients:

- Twenty strips of bacon (pasture-raised)
- Two avocados

Method:

1. Preheat your oven to 425 degrees Fahrenheit.
2. Take a baking sheet and line it with parchment
   paper.
3. Take the avocados and slice them in half
   lengthwise and remove their pits. Gently peel
   off the skin and slice the flesh of each avocado
   lengthwise into thin strips (five per half). Even
   though the flesh of the avocado is very soft, it
   stays stable without melting by holding up
   pretty well to the oven's high heat.
4. Wrap a strip of bacon around each slice of
   avocado and keep it on a parchment paper-
   lined baking sheet.
5. Keep it in the oven and allow it to cook for
   twenty-five to thirty minutes so that the bacon
   gets crisp. The cooking time depends on the
   slice of bacon. This recipe used thick-cut bacon.
   If you are using thinner cut bacon, it would

require ten minutes less to cook the bacon-wrapped avocado fries.
6. Allow them about five minutes to cool down before serving.
7. Serve them warm as a filling snack, game-day munchies, or a savory appetizer.

__Note__: Remember to choose pasture-raised pork when you are choosing your bacon. Pasture-raised pigs have a higher content of anti-inflammatory Omega-3 fatty acids and are naturally better for health.

Berry Popsicle

Total Prep & Cooking Time: 30 minutes + 6 hours
Yields: 12 servings
Nutrition Facts: Calories: 39 | Carbs: 9.8g | Protein: 0.4g | Fat: 0.2G | Fiber: 1.5G

Ingredients:

- Three cups each of
- Coconut water (unsweetened)
- Strawberries
- One and a half cups each of
- Blueberries
- Blackberries
- Two tablespoons of raw honey

Method:

1. In a blender, add 2 tsps. of raw honey, 1 cup of coconut oil, and blackberries and blend them together until you get a smooth paste.
2. Use a fine-mesh strainer to strain the mixture and eliminate the seeds of the blackberry. Keep this strained paste aside.
3. Repeat the above steps two more times with the blueberries and strawberries by utilizing one cup of coconut water and two tsp of honey for each flavor of berry.
4. Strain them using a fine-mesh strainer and keep them in separate bowls. Make sure to

keep all three strained flavors in separate
bowls.
5. Add the blueberry paste in the 1st third of your
Popsicle mold and keep it in the freezer until it
freezes and gets solid.
6. Repeat the previous step with the blackberry
and strawberry paste.
7. When you have finished filling the last berry
flavor into the popsicle molds, keep it in the
freezer for at least six hours or overnight.

*Note: In this recipe, a popsicle mold with loose sticks
that are secured in their place by the lid has been
used to make the berry popsicle. Remove the lid when
the strawberry layer has almost frozen and insert the
sticks into the almost frozen mixture. This way, you
will be able to fill up the last layer with the sticks still
in place. Although this might seem a bit tricky, it will
work just fine in the end.*

Chapter 6: Dessert Recipes

<u>*Banana Parfaits*</u>

Total Prep & Cooking Time: One hour and ten minutes
Yields: 3 servings
Nutrition Facts: Calories: 353.5 | Carbs: 71.2G |
Protein: 12.7G | Fat: 4.6g | Fiber: 6.8g

Ingredients:

For the pudding,
- Three bananas (ripe), divided
- One tablespoon of gelatin powder (unflavored)
- One 13.5 ounces of coconut milk (full-fat)
- One teaspoon of raw honey (optional)
- Half a teaspoon of vanilla extract (for AIP, use vanilla powder or omit)
- A dash each of
- Sea salt
- Turmeric (for some color of your liking)

For the cookie crumble,
- One-fourth of a cup of shredded coconut (unsweetened)
- Half a cup of coconut flour
- One tablespoon of maple syrup or raw honey
- One-fourth of a teaspoon of vanilla extract (for AIP, use sub-vanilla powder or omit)

- A sprinkle of cinnamon
- Four tablespoons of coconut oil
- A pinch of salt

Method:

1. In a medium-sized mixing bowl, add the coconut flour and gelatin and whisk them together until they are properly mixed. Allow it to rest or "bloom" for fifteen minutes.
2. Take the two bananas and mash them with the help of a fork (you should have about a cup of mashed bananas).
3. Add the mashed bananas into a high-speed blender along with the coconut milk and gelatin mixture, sea salt, vanilla essence, and turmeric powder. Blend them together for about twenty seconds or until they are combined properly.
4. Pour the pudding mixture into a bowl and cover it with a lid. Keep it in the refrigerator for at least an hour so that it sets.
5. Prepare the cookie crumb mixture in the meantime. For this, add the coconut flour, shredded coconut, raw honey or maple syrup, coconut oil, vanilla extract, cinnamon, and a pinch of salt in a food processor.
6. Spread the crumb on a baking sheet and allow it to bake in the oven for about ten to fifteen minutes until it turns golden brown in color.

7. Remove it from the oven once it turns golden brown and allow it to rest and come down to room temperature.
8. Cut the remaining banana into thin slices.
9. For layering the parfait, grab your serving cups and start by adding a layer of the cookie crumb, then some slices of bananas, followed by a layer of pudding and repeat.
10. You can finish it with whatever topping you like. You can add some more crumbs as the topping, or a sprinkle of cinnamon powder.

Chocolate Orange Truffles

Total Prep & Cooking Time: 5 hours and 30 minutes
Yields: 12 servings
Nutrition Facts: Calories: 158.6 | Carbs: 11.8g |
Protein: 1.5G | Fat: 12.4g | Fiber: 1.4g

Ingredients:

- One tablespoon of vegetable oil
- Eight squares of semi-sweet chocolate (about eight ounces), chopped
- One teaspoon of orange zest, grated
- Two tablespoons of orange liqueur
- Three tablespoons of heavy cream
- One-fourth of a cup of butter (unsalted)

Method:

1. Place a medium-sized saucepan over medium-high heat and add the heavy cream and butter into it. Combine them together and bring the mixture to a boil. Then, remove it from heat.
2. Add in the orange liqueur, orange zest, and four ounces of chopped chocolate into it and stir everything together until you get a smooth mixture.
3. Pour this truffle mixture into a 9-inch by 5-inch loaf pan or a shallow bowl. Chill it for about two hours so that it gets firm.
4. Take a baking sheet and line it with waxed paper. Using a rounded teaspoon or a melon

baller, shape the chilled truffle mixture and keep them on the prepared baking sheet. Allow them to chill for about thirty minutes so that they get firm.

5. Melt the remaining four ounces of semi-sweet chocolate with the vegetable oil in a double boiler placed over lightly simmering water and stir until it gets smooth. Let it cool down to lukewarm temperature.

6. Drop the truffles into the melted chocolate mixture one at a time. Take the truffles out of the chocolate using two forks. Before transferring them back onto the baking sheet, allow any extra chocolate to drip back into the pan. Let it chill until it sets.

Ginger Molasses Cookies

Total Prep & Cooking Time: Fifteen minutes
Yields: Ten servings
Nutrition Facts: Calories: 161 | Carbs: 11.8g | Protein: 3.4g | Fat: 12G | Fiber: 2.2G

Ingredients:

- One cup of almond flour
- One-fourth of a cup each of
- Coconut flour
- Coconut sugar
- Coconut oil, melted and cooled
- One egg, at room temperature
- Half a teaspoon each of
- Allspice
- Cinnamon
- Baking soda
- One-fourth of a teaspoon of salt
- Two tablespoons of molasses
- Three-fourth of a teaspoon of ground ginger
- One teaspoon of vanilla extract
- Organic sugar for rolling (optional)

Method:

1. Preheat your oven to 350 degrees Fahrenheit.
2. Mix together the egg, molasses, coconut sugar, vanilla extract, and the melted and cooled

coconut oil in a large bowl. Ensure that the
coconut oil is at room temperature.

3. Then, add the coconut flour, almond flour,
    baking soda, cinnamon, allspice, ground
    ginger, and salt into the bowl and mix
    everything properly so as to form a dough.
    Allow the dough to rest for a couple of minutes.
4. Scoop the dough using a cookie scoop and then
    roll the dough into balls using your hands.
5. Roll the dough balls in organic cane sugar if
    you want, and then keep them on an ungreased
    baking sheet. Using the back of a glass or your
    hands, gently flatten the dough.
6. Keep the baking sheet in the oven and allow the
    cookies to bake in the oven for about eight to
    eleven minutes.
7. After the cookies have finished baking, remove
    the baking sheet from the oven and allow the
    cookies to cool down on the baking sheet for
    about ten minutes before placing them on a
    wire rack to finish cooling.
8. This recipe makes about ten cookies, but feel
    free to double up the ingredients if you want
    more cookies.

Snack Mix

Total Prep & Cooking Time: 1 hour 15 minutes
Yields: 4 servings
Nutrition Facts: Calories: 130 | Carbs: 23G | Fat: 3.5g |
Fiber: 2G

Ingredients:

- One-fourth teaspoon salt
- Three tablespoons of coconut aminos
- Half tablespoon onion powder
- One tablespoon garlic powder
- One cup of dried cherries
- Four cups of coconut chips
- Four cups of plantain chips
- One-fourth cup and two tablespoons of coconut oil

Method:

1. At first, you need to preheat your oven to two hundred and fifty degrees.
2. Then you have to take a bowl and combine coconut flakes, cherries, and plantains. Stir well.
3. Then on low heat, melt coconut oil. Then you need to add salt, coconut aminos, onion powder, and garlic powder. Whisk.
4. Then take half of the snack mix and add it to the liquid. Then stir well for combining.

5. Then take the second half of the snack mix and add this too. Start stirring and continue until each and everything gets evenly coated.
6. Then you need to take the mixture and spread it on a cookie sheet or a roasting pan. Then place it in the oven for about an hour. Stir after every fifteen minutes.
7. Then when it is ready, keep the snack mix away for ten to fifteen minutes and allow it to cool down.

Coconut Jelly

Total Prep & Cooking Time: 15 minutes
Yields: 12 servings
Nutrition Facts: Calories: 216 | Carbs: 4g | Protein: 3g
| Fat: 19f | Fiber: 1G

Ingredients:

- Half teaspoon vanilla extract
- One teaspoon stevia (or any sweetener as per your choice)
- Twenty-seven ounces of coconut cream
- Half a cup of hot water
- Half a cup of water
- Two tablespoons of grass-fed gelatin

Method:

1. At first, you need to sprinkle some water on the gelatin for softening it for about one minute. Then you will have to add some hot water and stir so that it gets completely dissolved.
2. Then you have to take a medium-sized saucepan and pour some coconut cream. Then you have to turn the heat on medium and bring it to a slow boil.
3. Then to the saucepan, add the gelatin water. Then you need to cook for about five minutes. After five minutes, you need to remove the saucepan from heat. Then you have to add some vanilla extract and sweetener.

4. Then you need to pour this mixture into a
   baking dish. Finally, you have to leave it in the
   refrigerator until it is set.

Note: *For making the meal low on fat, you can use one can of coconut cream and one can of coconut milk. The coconut cream contributes to the flavor, so using only coconut milk is not recommended.*

**Raspberry Peppermint Bark**

Total Prep & Cooking Time: 55 minutes
Yields: 8 servings
Nutrition Facts: Calories: 144 | Carbs: 18g | Protein: 1.4g | Fat: 8.4g | Fiber: 0.7g

Ingredients:

- One-fourth cup of frozen, dried, and crushed raspberries
- One tablespoon filtered water
- One pinch salt
- Half cup of coconut concentrate
- Three teaspoons of peppermint extract
- One-fourth cup coconut oil
- Three tablespoons honey

Method:

1. At first, you have to turn on the heat on medium-low. Then you have to take a saucepan and add peppermint extract, coconut oil, and honey and heat it. Stir for combining them evenly. Then bring it to a simmer and then cook for about eight minutes accompanied by frequent stirring. Then you need to turn the heat down at the right time to prevent it from bubbling over.
2. Then you have to keep it aside for about fifteen minutes for allowing it to cool down.

3. After it gets cooled down, you need to put it into a food processor or a high powered blender along with the filtered water and the coconut concentrate. Then blend it on high speed until it gets fully blended. In case you observe a lack of consistency in the mixture, you can add more water (not more than one teaspoon at a time). Continue to add water and blend until you obtain a thick consistent paste.

4. Then take a small cookie sheet (or you can also use any other container that is flat enough and can easily fit inside a freezer), and pour the mixture onto it. The cookie sheet must be lined with parchment paper, and the mixture needs to be spread evenly with the help of a spatula. Then spread the paste in such a way that the layer has approximately one-fourth inch of thickness. Then on the top, sprinkle some raspberries, and then you need to gently press them down so that they get nicely stuck to the bark.

5. Then you have to keep it in the freezer and leave it there for about two hours to get set. Then you can use a knife to cut them into slices of any shape of your desire. Then you can store it inside any sort of sealed container and keep it inside a freezer or a refrigerator.

Peppermint Mocha Fudge

Total Prep & Cooking Time: 20 minutes
Yields: 12 servings
Nutrition Facts: Calories: 243 | Carbs: 21G | Protein: 3g | Fat: 16g | Fiber: 3g

Ingredients:

- One teaspoon salt
- Three tablespoons of maple syrup
- Half teaspoon peppermint extract
- One tablespoon instant coffee powder
- Half a cup of coconut milk
- Two and a half cups of semi-sweet chocolate chips

Method:

1. At first, take an eight by eight pan (or you can also use a nine by five-inch bread pan) and line it with parchment paper. Then you need to create a sling by allowing the parchment paper to go over the sides. Then you have to coat it lightly using a non-stick spray.
2. Then you have to take a small saucepan over medium-low heat. Then you need to add peppermint extract, maple syrup, instant coffee, coconut milk, and chocolate chips and allow them to melt. They will take about seven to twelve minutes to melt. Then you need to taste it and check the sweetness level and add

maple syrup accordingly (not more than one teaspoon at a time). Continue adding the maple syrup until your desired sweetness is reached. Then add one teaspoon salt.

3. Then the melted chocolate needs to be poured into your pan. Then you can top it with some more salt according to your taste.

4. Then you have to put it inside the refrigerator and keep it inside for a minimum of two hours. When it becomes firm, you have to take it out of the refrigerator and then cut it into small square slices. You can serve it either at room temperature, or you can also serve it cold.

Apple Crisp

Total Prep & Cooking Time: 1 hour
Yields: 6 servings
Nutrition Facts: Calories: 455 | Carbs: 44.5g | Protein:
2G | Fat: 31.8G | Fiber: 7.2G

Ingredients:

- Half a lemon's juice
- Two teaspoon cinnamon
- Three tablespoons of maple syrup
- One tablespoon tapioca starch
- One-fourth cup of softened coconut butter
- One-fourth cup of coconut flour
- One cup of shredded coconut
- One-third cup and two tablespoons of softened coconut oil
- Six peeled apples

Method:

1. At first, you need to preheat your oven to three hundred and seventy-five degrees.
2. Then you have to prepare the apples. Chop the apples into large square pieces and discard the core. Then take a bowl and pour the apple pieces. Then add half a lemon's juice, cinnamon, and two tablespoons of coconut oil and combine them. Take an eight by eight

inches baking sheet and scoop the apples into it. Then keep it aside.

3. Then for making the crisp, take a bowl and add tapioca starch, coconut flour, and shredded coconut and mix them well. Then add maple syrup, coconut butter, and one-third cup of coconut oil. Mix them well.

4. Then use your hands and evenly spread the crisp mixture onto the apples. Push downwards for spreading out.

5. Bake it for about 40 to 45 minutes in the oven, until the crisp turns golden brown in color.

6. You can either serve it as it is or can also serve it with ice cream.

Carob Pudding

Total Prep time: Five minutes
Yields: Three servings
Nutrition Facts: Calories: 246 | Carbs: 43.2 | Protein: 3.8g | Fat: 7.7g | Fiber: 3.6g

Ingredients:

- Two avocados
- One-third cup of carob powder
- Half a tsp. of the vanilla extract
- Two tbsp. of maple syrup
- One tbsp. of coconut oil

Method:

1. Scoop out the avocado's flesh into the blender. Add all ingredients to the bowl of the blender and blend it on high speed until you notice a smooth and silky texture.
2. Serve it immediately. You may even store it inside the refrigerator for two days and enjoy the chilled pudding.

Note: *This is rich in its taste and very satisfying though it is barely sweet. You will be able to feel the avocado's creaminess, and adding the salt to it brings all the taste together and gives you a really yummy and delicious pudding.*

Apple Cinnamon Bars

Total Prep & cooking Time: 55 minutes
Yields: Twelve bars
Nutrition Facts: Calories: 120 | Carbs: 24g | Protein: 2G | Fat: 3g | Fiber: 3g

Ingredients:

- Half a cup each of
- Tiger nut flour
- Tiger nuts (sliced)
- Raisins
- One tablespoon each of
- Maple syrup
- Collagen hydrolysate
- One-third cup of unsweetened coconut (organic and shredded)
- One teaspoon each of
- Cinnamon
- Seal salt
- One riced plantain (ripe)
- Coconut or avocado oil (for greasing)
- One small-sized apple (cored, shredded, peeled)
- A quarter teaspoon of clove (ground)

Method:

1. Set your oven at a temperature of 350 degrees F. Then keep it preheated, and while doing this, use a bowl to mix together tiger nut flour,

coconut, tiger nuts, raisins, cinnamon, clove, salt, and collagen. Mix them well, and to this mixture, add the apple, maple syrup, and the riced plantain. Combine them well so that they get incorporated.

2. You will require a baking dish that has a dimension of 8x8 inches. Grease it using oil and then lay down the mixture on it evenly. Bake this mixture for about thirty minutes.

3. Take it out and allow it to settle in for some time, and by this time, it will get cooled. Cut it into pieces and enjoy.

Oatmeal Raisin Cookies

Total Prep & Cooking Time: 30 minutes
Yields: Fourteen cookies
Nutrition Facts: Calories: 156 | Carbs: 12G | Protein: 3g | Fat: 11G | Fiber: 1G

Ingredients:

- One and a quarter cups of almond flour (blenched)
- Half a teaspoon each of
- Vanilla extract (pure)
- Baking soda
- A quarter cup each of
- Tapioca flour
- Almond butter (smooth and unsalted)
- Maple syrup (pure)
- Coconut oil (soft and solid), it is better to use refined oil to avoid the smell of coconut
- A quarter teaspoon of salt
- Half a cup of raisins
- A three-fourth teaspoon of cinnamon

One flax egg: To prepare this egg, you will require one tablespoon of flaxseed (ground) and two and a half tbsp. of water. Mix the two of them and allow them to settle for about ten to fifteen minutes.

Method:

1. Before you can start with this recipe, you will have to prepare the flax egg, and for that, you will have to go through the ingredients section thoroughly. The preparation of the flax egg is already given there.

2. Set your oven at a temperature of 350 degrees Fahrenheit. Allow it to heat up and keep it preheated.

3. Take a bowl where you can mix the almond, baking soda, cinnamon, tapioca flour, and salt. Whisk them properly and then keep it aside for use later.

4. In the second bowl, add coconut oil and almond butter. Mix them with the help of a mixer (preferably an electric one) to form a smooth paste. In between the processing, add maple syrup and the vanilla. After adding these, again continue with the mixer until the whole thing becomes perfectly smooth. Beat in the flax egg to combine fully. The beating of the egg must be done slowly and not at all in a hurry!

5. The batter is now ready to be added into the flour mixture. Add the flours using small scoops and combine it thoroughly to form cookie dough that is fairly sticky. Drop the raisins and fold into the dough and allow them to settle for about five minutes.

6. Now it is the time to remove the cookie dough to a sheet (for placing cookie) with the help of a scoop. The measurement of the scoop must be that of a tablespoon. So, scoop them out and

then place them on the baking sheet at about a distance of two inches.

7. Place them in the already heated oven and bake for fifteen minutes. This time is enough to make their edges brown with a soft center. It is completely okay if they are soft instead of having a chewy texture.

8. After removing from the oven, let them cool down for five minutes over the wire rack. This amount of dough will form nearly fourteen cookies. Serve and enjoy.

Almond Flour Brownies

Total Prep & Cooking Time: 25 minutes
Yields: Eight servings
Nutrition Facts: Calories: 189 | Carbs: 13.4g | Protein: 3.8g | Fat: 14.7g | Fiber: 2.8g

Ingredients:

- A quarter cup of coconut oil
- One tsp. of vanilla extract
- A two-third cup of almond flour
- One-eighth tsp. of baking soda
- Twelve raspberries
- One-third cup of coconut sugar
- One egg kept at room temperature
- Three tbsp. of cocoa powder (unsweetened)
- A quarter tsp. of salt

For the drizzle,
- A quarter tsp. of coconut oil
- Two tbsp. of chocolate chips (vegan) or dairy-free

Method:

1. Set the oven at a temperature of 350 degrees F and preheat. The two different ways in which these brownies are possible to make are - the first way is to use a loaf pan, and the second way is to use two small-sized skillets.

2. In case you are using the skillets, then you will
    require two of them, each measuring five
    inches and generously grease them with
    coconut oil. And a loaf pan, if preferred, should
    be of the dimension 8x4 inch and lined with a
    parchment paper.
3. Turn the flame of the oven to low and place the
    saucepan over it. To the saucepan, add the
    coconut sugar and coconut oil. After adding,
    stir the oil in a way that it melts fully, and the
    combination becomes shiny. Set the mixture
    away, allowing it to cool down, and after it has
    been cooled, remove it to a bowl that is
    medium in size. To this bowl, you may add
    vanilla extract and the eggs. Whisk them
    completely to make a paste. The batter thus
    prepared must be a smooth one.
4. In this step, you will be adding the dry
    ingredients to the batter - cocoa powder, salt,
    almond flour, and the baking soda. Stir them
    thoroughly to form a smooth mixture. This
    time the prepared batter will be thick. Spread
    the thickened batter either in the skillets or in
    the pan evenly—Crown the brownie batter with
    the raspberries by pushing them inside it
    gently.
5. While baking in skillets, allow the batter to
    bake for about fifteen minutes so that the
    margins of the brownie pull themselves away
    from the sides. And in a loaf pan, the required
    time for the brownie to bake will be twenty-

three minutes, which will be enough to set the brownies in shape.

6. Allowing the brownies to stay fudgy is usually recommended.
7. Remove the brownies to a rack made of wire whose main purpose is to make them cool.
8. *Preparing the chocolate drizzle*: Cook the chocolate chips in coconut oil over low heat. After making them smooth, drizzle them over the laid brownies. Serve them on the serving plate.

Fudgy Pumpkin Brownies

Total Prep & Cooking Time: 30 minutes
Yields: Twelve brownies
Nutrition Facts: Calories: 135 | Carbs: 15.3G | Protein: 3.4g | Fat: 8.2G | Fiber: 3.4g

Ingredients:

- Three-fourth cup each of
- Puree of pumpkin
- Almond flour
- One-third cup of maple syrup (pure)
- One tsp. of vanilla extract
- Three tbsp. of coconut flour
- Two eggs
- Half a tsp. each of
- Baking soda
- Cinnamon
- Baking powder
- One-third cup of cocoa powder (unsweetened)
- A quarter tsp. each of
- Allspice
- Salt
- A quarter cup of chips of chocolate

For the topping,
- One tsp. of coconut oil
- Two tbsp. of chocolate chips

Method:

1. Set your oven at a temperature of 350 degrees
    F. Then keep it preheated. You will prepare
    these brownies in a pan and therefore use a
    parchment paper for bordering it.
2. You will need a large-sized bowl to mix the
    vanilla extract, maple syrup, pumpkin puree,
    and the eggs. Whisk the eggs properly to make
    the batter smooth.
3. To this bowl, add all the dry ingredients -
    almond flour, cocoa powder, allspice, baking
    soda, cinnamon, baking powder, salt, and
    coconut flour. Whip them together to form a
    smooth paste.
4. To this batter, fold in a quarter cup of chocolate
    chips.
5. Pour the batter that was prepared inside the
    bowl into the parchment-lined pan. After it is
    poured, make the top of the batter smooth with
    the help of a spatula. Bake the batter for about
    twenty-five minutes. You will know that the
    brownie is baked after a knife once inserted
    into the brownie comes off clean. It might look
    as if the brownies are not cooked fully, but a
    clear knife would mean that they are all done.
    Transfer the brownies to a rack and keep them
    for fifteen minutes to cool.
6. *Preparation of the chocolate paste*: You will
    have to place a saucepan in the oven over low
    heat and pour the coconut oil into it. Drop the
    chips into the saucepan and stir to make a
    smooth paste. Cut the brownie into twelve

pieces, and over each of them, drizzle the melted chocolate to form the topping.

**Maple Walnut Sugar Cookies**

Total Prep & Cooking Time: 25 minutes
Yields: Fourteen cookies
Nutrition Facts: Calories: 168.97 | Carbs: 5.25g |
Protein: 4.76g | Fat: 15.51G | Fiber: 2.12G

Ingredients:

For the dough of cookie,
- A quarter cup each of
- Maple syrup (pure) or coconut sugar
- Coconut oil
- One egg which is kept at room temperature
- Half a teaspoon each of
- Sea salt (fine grain)
- Baking soda
- One teaspoon of vanilla extract (pure)
- Two cups of almond flour (blenched)
- A three-fourth cup of walnuts, chopped

For the maple glaze,
- Half a cup of maple sugar (powdered)
- Half a teaspoon of vanilla
- Two teaspoons of almond milk

Method:

1. Set your oven at a temperature of 350 degrees
   F. Then keep the oven preheated. For baking

these cookies, you will require a baking sheet, and for that, line it with a parchment paper.

2. Take a large-sized bowl. In this bowl, add the coconut oil or ghee, maple syrup, vanilla, egg, and maple sugar. Whisk these ingredients together in order to form a smooth mixture.

3. In another bowl, add almond flour, salt, and baking soda. These ingredients must be whipped completely to form a mixture. Now, in this bowl, stir in the dry ingredients mixture that was prepared in the first bowl until it forms a sticky dough. Finally, add in the walnuts (chopped).

4. Cover the bowl and keep it inside the refrigerator. Allow it to stay inside for about twenty minutes. A medium-sized cookie scoop measuring about one and a half tablespoon will be enough to scoop out the dough. After scooping the dough pieces out, place them on the baking sheet maintaining a two inches distance among each of them because the cookies will spread after they are baked.

5. Place them in the oven that was preheated for about twelve minutes until they become golden brown. Take them out of the oven and let them settle to cool down by not disturbing them for ten minutes. After they are cooled, transfer them to the rack where they will be cooled down completely.

6. *Preparation of the glaze*: Meanwhile, you can mix the maple sugar (powdered), vanilla, and almond milk to form a paste of a consistency

that it can be drizzled. In case the mixture becomes too thick, add some drops of almond milk.

7. After the glaze has been prepared, pour it over the cookies (the cookies must have cooled down by then). Allow the glaze to settle over the cookies for about twenty minutes. Serve them and enjoy.

If you enjoyed this book, please let me know your thoughts by leaving a short review on Amazon. Thank you!

Conclusion

Thank you for making it through to the end of *Autoimmune Diet for Beginners*, let's hope it was informative and able to provide you with all of the tools you need to achieve your goals whatever they may be.

It is completely okay if you are not an expert in cooking because not everyone is a gourmet chef, and that is why the recipes that I have included in this book are extremely easy to make. Even if you have limited experience in the kitchen, you shouldn't be having any problem making these. I simply want to remind you of one small thing – the autoimmune diet is meant to support your body to maintain a strong immune system. It does not, in any way, replace routine health care.

But I am confident that if you are going to follow this diet for an extended period of time, it will improve your overall health. But never think that this diet is a cure-all. It is just one of the several tools you can put in your toolbox to keep yourself healthy. There are so many things that you still need to take care of. For example, you have to ensure that you are sleeping on time, and your body feels restful and energetic when you wake up. You also need to drink sufficient amount of water every day. You have to do some kind of exercise to raise the metabolism levels in your body and you also need to find ways in which you can relieve stress. This can be something as simple as deep breathing exercises or a daily ritual like yoga. You have to select something that works best for you. And lastly, if you have any health concern, don't wait for this diet to do any magic because, like I said before, this diet is only meant to support your body's immune system. If you have some underlying problem, you have to see a licensed health practitioner or a doctor.

"Other books by Alexander Great"

Autoimmune Protocol Diet: *The Complete Guide to the Protocol to Improving Your Health With the Autoimmune Diet: https://www.amazon.com/dp/B08D2J6V37*

Autoimmune Diet Cookbook: *Complete Step-By-Step Guide to Cooking Healthy Dishes and Increase Immune Defenses With The Autoimmune Solution: https://www.amazon.com/dp/B08D3Y66G7*

Autoimmune Disease Anti-Inflammatory Diet: *30 Healthy Anti-Inflammatory Recipes to Eat Well Every Day and Improve Health Fast Without Feeling on a Diet: https://www.amazon.com/dp/B08CYB3WWQ*

AIP Diet : *4 Manuscripts: Autoimmune Protocol Diet, Autoimmune Disease Anti-Inflammatory Diet, Autoimmune Diet for Beginners, Autoimmune Diet Cookbook https://www.amazon.com/dp/B08JWP59MD*